The Patient and Health Care System: Perspectives on High-Quality Care

Pranavi V. Sreeramoju • Stephen G. Weber
Alexis A. Snyder • Lynne M. Kirk
William G. Reed • Beverly A. Hardy-Decuir
Editors

The Patient and Health Care System: Perspectives on High-Quality Care

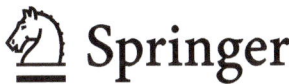 Springer

Editors
Pranavi V. Sreeramoju
Department of Internal Medicine
UT Southwestern Medical Center
Dallas
TX
USA

Alexis A. Snyder
Independent Engagement Specialist and
Patient Family Advisor
Brookline
MA
USA

William G. Reed
Quality, Safety and Outcomes Education
UT Southwestern Medical Center
Dallas
TX
USA

Stephen G. Weber
The University of Chicago Medicine
Chicago
IL
USA

Lynne M. Kirk
Department of Internal Medicine
UT Southwestern Medical Center
Dallas
TX
USA

Beverly A. Hardy-Decuir
Quality and Clinical Effectiveness
Parkland Health and Hospital System
Dallas
TX
USA

ISBN 978-3-030-46566-7   ISBN 978-3-030-46567-4   (eBook)
https://doi.org/10.1007/978-3-030-46567-4

This Springer imprint is published by the registered company Springer Nature Switzerland AG
The registered company address is: Gewerbestrasse 11, 6330 Cham, Switzerland

Introduction

In health care, we are humans taking care of other humans. Patients place their trust and their lives and money in the health care system, counting on us to treat their illnesses and help them get healthier. Health care professionals have different roles, as physicians, nurses, administrators, quality and safety professionals, policy experts, lawmakers, and researchers, to name a few, and for the most part, they are united by an overarching desire to heal, provide care, and save lives.

This book is about the interface between the patient and the health care system, where, as they say, the rubber meets the road. This interface between the patient and the health care system is an extremely complicated place where all the good intentions, expertise, and actions come together. In spite of the existing knowledge on achieving health care quality and high-value care, oftentimes we have trouble defining what we should aim for in health care, what our true north is. The metrics we have in place to measure quality, safety, and value do not do sufficient justice to what we seem to be looking for, as professionals, consumers, and stakeholders. If we aim to provide high-quality care that is accessible, affordable, and equitable for everyone, then we ought to have a more inclusive conversation on how to improve health care delivery.

In this book, we have a series of diverse voices and perspectives from those who strive to improve health care delivery and dedicated their careers to the same. This book is written keeping in mind those who have a stake in improving health care. One could easily argue that it includes everyone. The authors built on ongoing conversations and solutions in health care and presented original, creative, and thought-provoking perspectives that go way beyond how topics in quality, safety, and value in health care have been historically treated. The chapters have great diversity in content, style, and perspective, and each stands alone by itself. Readers can elect to read the chapters either in random order or cover to cover. While some authors specifically included a call for action to patients, physicians, nurses, administrators, payers, and policymakers, everyone universally has challenged the reader to reflect more and engage more in solving the problem of health care in a meaningful and reasonable manner. The main goal is for the reader to think about how s/he can contribute to how we solve the problem of health care, which right now is bigger than the solutions we have been able to come up with thus far. There are many individuals who would not be alive or healthy today if not for our state-of-the-art health care system. Yet, it is also true that our health care system has failed some individuals in one way or another. Because of where the authors live and work, this book is about health care systems in the United States. However, many principles apply to health care systems everywhere in the world.

If the topic of the book sounds complicated, it is because it is. Hence, this book hopes to target key issues at stake and nudge us towards potential actions that each of us can take.

Finally, we would like to highlight the connections among people with diverse professional interests that made this book possible. This book may not have begun if Nadina Persaud from Springer Publishing had not approached Pranavi V. Sreeramoju for a book idea. Pranavi V. Sreeramoju in turn reached out to Alexis Snyder, Stephen Weber, Lynne Kirk, Gary Reed, and Beverly Hardy-Decuir with the book idea and together they shaped the focus and scope of the book. Pranavi V. Sreeramoju uses her training and experience in infectious diseases, health care epidemiology, and, more recently, quality and finance to help improve health care delivery for patients in a large academic medical center and blogs to increase awareness on issues in health care. Stephen Weber has expertise in infectious diseases and health care epidemiology and is a strong advocate for greater leadership in health care delivery improvement as reflected in his chapter on the voice of the physician as well as the epilogue. Alexis Snyder is Patient Family Advisor and Engagement Specialist who is a relentless advocate for making health care delivery as well as outcomes research more patient-centered and more inclusive of the patient and family voice.

Gary Reed led health system quality efforts for many years and currently leads medical school colleges as well as education on quality and safety at a large academic medical center. Lynne Kirk has a wealth of experience in medical education, patient-centered care, and leadership in organized medicine. Last, but not the least, Beverly Hardy-Decuir contributes rich experiences as a nurse and a professional in quality. Each of the authors were identified through existing connections, and they wrote the chapters with the sole motivation of sharing their thoughts and ideas on how to improve health care delivery and received no material compensation for their contributions. Each author's personal and professional experiences with health care are in some way reflected in the chapters. This book is a collective attempt to frame the conversation and use our connections to improve health care delivery. We are thankful to Dhanapal Palanisamy, ArulRonika Pathinathan, Henry Rodgers and Cecily Berberat for their assistance with production and development of the book and to our families for sparing some family time to let us put this together.

Contents

Contributors

Debra Albert, DNP, MBA, RN, NEA-BC The University of Chicago Medicine, Chicago, IL, USA

David J. Ballard, MD, MSPH, PhD Department of Health Policy and Management, UNC Gillings School of Public Health, The University of North Carolina at Chapel Hill, Chapel Hill, NC, USA

Eugene S. Chu, MD UT Southwestern Division of Hospital Medicine at Parkland Hospital, Department of Internal Medicine, UT Southwestern Medical Center, Dallas, TX, USA

Briget da Graca, JD, MS Baylor Scott & White Research Institute, Dallas, TX, USA

Robbins Institute for Health Policy and Leadership, Hankamer School of Business, Baylor University, Waco, TX, USA

Lucía Durá, PhD Department of English, The University of Texas at El Paso, El Paso, TX, USA

Neil S. Fleming, PhD Robbins Institute for Health Policy and Leadership, Hankamer School of Business, Baylor University, Waco, TX, USA

Stephen J. Harder, MD UT Southwestern Division of Hospital Medicine at Parkland Hospital, Department of Internal Medicine, UT Southwestern Medical Center, Dallas, TX, USA

Beverly A. Hardy-Decuir, DNP, MSN, FACHE, CPHQ Quality and Clinical Effectiveness, Parkland Health and Hospital System, Dallas, TX, USA

Krista Hirschmann, PhD, FAACH Academy of Communication in Health Care, Allentown, PA, USA

Lynne M. Kirk, MD Department of Internal Medicine, UT Southwestern Medical Center, Dallas, TX, USA

Department of Accreditation Services, Accreditation Council for Graduate Medical Education, Chicago, IL, USA

Keith Kosel, PhD, MHSA, MBA Population Health Group, Parkland Center for Clinical Innovation, Dallas, TX, USA

Jessica Mantel, JD, MPP University of Houston Law Center, Houston, TX, USA

Donna Persaud, MD, MBA Population Health, Parkland Health and Hospital System, Dallas, TX, USA

William G. Reed, MD Department of Internal Medicine, UT Southwestern Medical Center, Dallas, TX, USA

Quality, Safety and Outcomes Education, UT Southwestern Medical Center, Dallas, TX, USA

Sheira Schlair, MD, MS Department of Medicine, Montefiore Medical Center, Einstein College of Medicine, Bronx, NY, USA

John Jay Shannon, MD Department of Medicine, Cook County Health, Chicago, IL, USA

Alexis A. Snyder, BA Independent Engagement Specialist and Patient Family Advisor, Brookline, MA, USA

Pranavi V. Sreeramoju, MD, MPH, MBA Department of Internal Medicine, UT Southwestern Medical Center, Dallas, TX, USA

Sally Walton, MSN, MBA, RN, OCN, NEA-BC The University of Chicago Medicine, Chicago, IL, USA

Stephen G. Weber, MD, MS Professor of Medicine, Chief Medical Officer and Senior Vice President for Clinical Excellence, The University of Chicago Medicine, Chicago, IL, USA

Part I

Voices

Voice of the Patient

1

Alexis A. Snyder

> *The human voice is the most beautiful instrument of all, but it is the most difficult to play* [1]
>
> —*Richard Strauss*

"Nothing for Us without Us"

A powerful phrase that can be heard from patients, family members, and patient advocates all across our nation. But what exactly does this mean? Let's first take a closer look at the definition of patient-centeredness. While there may be multiple ways to describe patient-centered care, the National Academy of Medicine defines patient-centered care as, "Providing care that is respectful of, and responsive to, individual patient preferences, needs and values, and ensuring that patient values guide all clinical decisions [2]." To respond to this definition, health care systems have a responsibility to identify what those preferences, needs, and values are, and what is most important to whom, when, and under what circumstances. But how can health care systems achieve this surmountable task? The answer is both simple and complex: ask the patient.

When we talk about patient-centeredness, it only makes sense that the patient, who is at the center of the care, be included in all aspects of their care. After all, systems can't practice "patient-centeredness" without the "patient." Patients need to have a voice in the systems that affect the care they receive. But often the patient voice goes unheard. Perhaps because they are afraid to speak up, or too ill and/or devoid of the energy to participate in their care. Maybe there is a cultural piece at play, or a belief system that the professionals know best. Perhaps the patient is skilled at self-advocacy, but systems are not in place to incorporate their voice.

A. A. Snyder (✉)
Independent Engagement Specialist and Patient Family Advisor, Brookline, MA, USA

P. V. Sreeramoju et al. (eds.), *The Patient and Health Care System: Perspectives on High-Quality Care*, https://doi.org/10.1007/978-3-030-46567-4_1

Whether the patient and their caregivers are willing and able to share their voices or not, the health care system must empower their voices and allow them to come to the forefront. We cannot determine what is most important to patients and families when we don't ask.

The patient voice is vital to understanding the individual needs of the patient in the clinical setting and even more crucial to determining if the programs and services delivered to patients and families work, and for whom and when. We all know the saying… "the best laid plans…" and how this sentence ends. We can incorporate this into health care and patient engagement. Health systems cannot run on assumptions about what patients want. Clinicians, administrators, and health care systems may have the best of intentions when planning and implementing services for patients, but without patient input into these structures and designs, systems may fail at meeting patients' needs, thereby increasing costs. Patient engagement in health care can improve the effectiveness and efficiency of services received. Hospitals that engage patients in care have reduced lengths of stays, decreased adverse events, and even high employee retention rates [3]. Patient and family involvement in decision-making has been associated in primary care settings with improved health status and increased efficiency of care [4].

Incorporating the Patient and Family Voice

How to best incorporate the patient and family voice in health care is often seen as a challenge. How to gather information and include it in practice change and improvement can vary by institution. To understand how to include the patient voice, it's important to first understand that "patient voice" goes beyond the patient and can include family members, caregivers, and even the larger community. Hearing all these voices, and bringing them to the table, has been a long process over the last two decades. Let's take a brief look at some of the milestones that brought the patient voice into health care. Let's start with Patient and Family Advisory Councils, otherwise known as PFACs, which comprise patients, family, and staff members who work together to improve the patient experiences, and help implement change.

In 1998, Dana-Farber Cancer Institute in Boston, Massachusetts, incepted one of the first ever Patient and Family Advisory Councils, which became the national model for health care institutions to create PFACs and, therefore, improve the patient experience and ensure patient- and family-centered care [5]. In 2006, the World Health Organization (WHO) created a specific program area within their Patient Safety Program called Patients for Patient Safety [6]. That same year, a Massachusetts statewide consumer health advocacy organization, Health Care for All, in Boston, Massachusetts, organized the Consumer Health Quality Council to advocate for health legislation that ensured Massachusetts health care consumers receive health care that is, "efficient, effective, timely, safe, and patient-centered [7]." For the next 2 years, the council worked on legislation to advocate for an omnibus health care quality improvement bill that led to a number of provisions of the bill becoming law. One of which included a law, enacted in 2008, which required all

Massachusetts hospitals to create and maintain a PFAC. This was followed by a regulation enacted in 2009, from the Massachusetts Department of Public Health (DPH), regarding all Massachusetts hospitals to establish a PFAC by 2010 [8]. As of 2015, there were 97 hospital PFACs across Massachusetts [9], a standard that has set an example and helped the growth of PFACs nationwide. During this same time, the WHO developed a formal position that defines patient and family engagement as, "essential for patient safety and quality improvement efforts [6]."

Today, PFACs are a well-recognized best practice, not only in the hospital setting but in primary care as well, with many systems implementing patient-specific councils in different disciplines such as Pediatrics and Behavioral Health. With agencies such as the WHO, Health Care for All, and others beginning to emphasize the importance of partnering with patients for quality improvement efforts, the role of patients and families began to take on a new meaning, while empowered to use their voices and share their perspectives in a unique way.

Achieving Authentic Engagement

Implementing a PFAC is a move toward patient-centeredness, but it alone does not make a hospital or health care setting patient-centered. To be truly patient-centered, health systems must authentically and fully engage patients and families. Adding a patient and family advisory council shouldn't just check a box on list, or invite patients to weigh in on mundane tasks, such as choosing new paint colors for a waiting area, or providing feedback on the quality of the food and menu choices. While these less meaningful tasks can serve a purpose, they alone do not fully engage patients and allow the health systems to fully utilize, and recognize, the valuable contributions of patients. Partnering with patients to their full potential, in meaningful ways, allows their voices to positively impact program and policy decisions that affect the care they and others receive. Some systems are very good at incorporating the patient voice into planning and development, and implementation and evaluation, while others are still learning. When I think about these inconsistencies in practice, I am reminded of a phrase coined by my daughter's physical therapist to describe the fluctuations in her neuromuscular system, "consistently inconsistent." "Consistently Inconsistent" seems an appropriate term for how health systems engage patients.

Inconsistencies over how to incorporate the patient voice often exist over confusion between patient engagement and patient experience. Patient experience is defined by the Beryl Institute as, "the sum of all interactions, shaped by an organization's culture, that influence patient perceptions across the continuum of care [10]." In other words, the perception of what the patient is experiencing with every encounter with the health system, be it a phone call, an office visit, and so forth. Every encounter is affected by interactions with staff and providers. Patient engagement can be defined as "patients working in active partnership at various levels across the health care system to improve health and health care [11]." To be truly engaged, the patient must actively participate in their own health care, and/or work to improve the experience for others.

Here we can see how the two concepts, experience and engagement, go hand in hand. When a patient has a poor experience or encounter with the health care system, they may no longer engage. Without engaging, the patient cannot help improve the experience for themselves or for others in the future. Both patient engagement and patient experience play an important role in incorporating the patient voice. Both are necessary to make health systems patient-centered, and components of each are associated with "making it work" for the patient. Yet, often, systems rely on only patient experience measures, such as HCAHPS (Hospital Consumer Assessment of Health Care Providers and Systems) scores [12], to evaluate how the system is engaging patients, and this is where it goes wrong. Measuring patient experience alone does not fully engage patients, and the two are absolutely dependent on each other. Without evaluating the experience of the patient, systems cannot determine where improvement is needed and where to engage patients in process improvement efforts.

Achieving success in patient satisfaction and process improvement relies on both measuring experience and employing active engagement, both of which require the patient voice. The differences between passive and active engagement also play a role in effective communication in engagement. Passive engagement doesn't necessarily require the presence of patients, and is more about measuring patient experience, such as participating in an online survey. Active engagement, however, requires the presence of patients to interact with the system and to engage with available resources to promote change. So how do health systems include the patient voice and achieve authentic engagement? First let's take a look at what I will call the three "E's".

Empower, Engage, and Emplace

Empower patients to take an active role in their own health care. Rather than ask questions that passively engage the patient, such as "How do you feel?" or "How was your visit?", ask patient-centered questions that promote active engagement, such as "How can I best help?" and "What can we do differently?" Support patients and their families by valuing what they have to say. If you are going to ask what is most important to them, be ready to hear the answer. When patients feel respected and listened to, they feel empowered to actively participate in their own care. Empower patients to advocate for themselves, and if they are able for others, so that they may help make the experience for others more positive. Create a supportive environment where patients and their caregivers can be listened to without being judged and are valued for what they have to offer. When patients feel valued for their opinion, they realize they have a voice that can be used to make a difference for others as well. Listen to what the patient or family member is telling you; truly listen. Don't dismiss concerns over symptoms. Patients are the experts of their bodies; providers are the experts of medicine; work together. Providers and health care systems can best help patients in their times of need when patients, as well as their caregivers, are fully included in decision-making. Collaborate with patients 1:1

through shared decision-making to promote autonomy, and consistency with treatments, while creating stronger and more confident patients who have a voice in, and some control over, their own health. Believability and trust go a long way. It is very difficult to imagine what someone else is going through when it doesn't directly affect us. As the old saying goes, "You can't understand someone until you've walked a mile in their shoes." This is why we truly need to listen to patient stories, learn from them, and ask how we can improve next time. And this goes for patients of all ages, even children.

Samantha,[1] age 11, loved to read. She would read book after book, sometimes for hours at a time. Then one day, she stopped reading. Not only did she stop reading for fun, she stopped reading for homework too. Already under the care of an ophthalmologist for other medical reasons, her mother scheduled an appointment for Samantha. At the appointment, Samantha received a clean bill of eye health. Samantha informed the doctor that she was having some difficulty reading. The doctor who had just given Samantha a brief vision test, seemed surprised. She stated "I don't see any medical reason for that" and "You are too young to be needing reading glasses." Samantha still insisted she could not see the words on a page well, but her voice went unanswered. With her mother's persistence, the doctor did one more vision test. Nothing new was revealed, and the doctor was ready to send Samantha home telling her mother "there is nothing wrong with her vision, it's likely an excuse to not complete her homework."

Knowing this was not the case, Samantha's mother persisted again, pointing out that Samantha loves to read, has stopped, and there must be a reason. The doctor hesitated for a moment, but then suggested Samantha might like to see a specialized optometrist who could perhaps provide some exercises to help eye fatigue, but she was not sure it would make a difference. A couple of weeks later, Samantha was seen by the optometrist, who uncovered that Samantha's eyes were having difficulty converting between seeing at a distance and then up close; she diagnosed Samantha with Convergence Insufficiency, a disorder in which the eyes are unable to work together to look at nearby objects, causing double or blurred vision; something that isn't typically detected in routine eye exams or vision screenings [13].

Samantha received an eyeglass prescription that allowed her eye muscles to relax and enable them to more easily adjust between near and far, and soon thereafter she was enjoying reading again. Sometimes health problems are not obvious, as was the case with Samantha. There is a metaphor in the patient world that says, "When you hear hoof beats, don't assume to find a horse, you just might find a zebra." In other words, don't assume the obvious, and take the time to think outside the box, because even though it might sound like a horse, it might actually be a zebra.

Good doctor-patient relationships foster positive experiences that lead to positive engagement. Relationships with a health system actually start before the patient even walks through the door. It starts with the first person the patient has contact with and, if we are talking about an outpatient visit, for example, the first point of

[1] The patients' stories in this chapter are based on real-life events, only the names of the patients have been changed to protect their privacy.

contact is likely with a support person over the phone. After that, the experience continues with the front line staff at the appointment. This interaction can actually make or break an appointment. If the patient has a poor experience with the phone support or the front line staff in person, no matter how much the patient likes the provider, it may still reflect negatively on the overall experience, leaving the patient to consider going elsewhere, where they may feel more respected. It's no coincidence that "hospital" can be found in the word "hospitality," which by definition means "the quality or disposition of receiving and treating guests and strangers in a warm, friendly, generous way [14]." While this is sometimes hard to do, it must be done to establish a good rapport with the patient. No matter how much the patient values the provider, the value can be diminished, and as we learned earlier, poor experience can lead to poor empowerment, and poor engagement.

Engage. What does engagement mean to you? One good definition to consider is "A mutually beneficial interaction that results in participants feeling valued for their unique contribution [15]." If we use this definition, how can we apply this to patients and their interaction with the health care system? The answer is start with engaging patients, caregivers, and the larger community often and in meaningful ways. Create an atmosphere of trust and value what patients and families have to offer. Collaborate with patients to their fullest potential by engaging them in activities that make a real difference; activities that rely on the patient perspective to support and enhance the goals and outcomes of the project, as well as the overarching goals of the health system—a unique contribution that is "mutually beneficial."

If we think about active versus passive engagement, and apply it to this definition, we may really be defining authentic engagement as moving across a path from low involvement or inclusion, to high engagement and partnership. This spectrum of engagement can be looked at on a continuum from low level, where patients are involved by merely informing them, to a high level of engagement where systems partner with patients to achieve a mutually beneficial interaction. This continuum of engagement has been defined by Health Canada, the department of the government of Canada with responsibility for national public health [16], as part of their tool kit for public involvement in decision-making [17], and it can easily be applied to achieving authentic patient and family engagement (Fig. 1.1).

This model of involvement and decision-making gives us a clear framework that helps explain the difference between involvement and engagement and how both have a place in how health system decisions are made, to what degree the patient voice is able to have an influence, and how much influence on those decisions and, ultimately, on outcomes. We can also use this spectrum of engagement to define whether health systems and providers are delivering services TO patients, FOR patients, or WITH patients, a concept more simply known as *TO FOR WITH*.

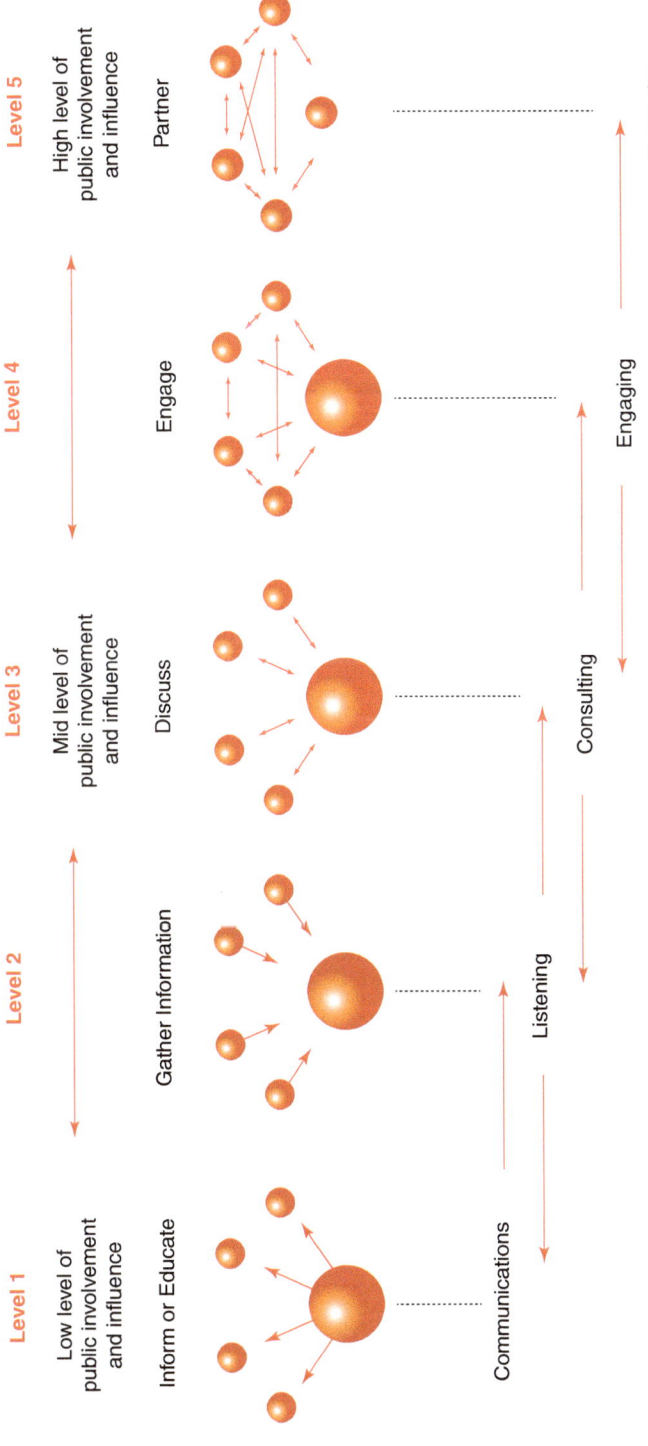

Fig. 1.1 Health Canada's public involvement continuum. (Adapted from Patterson Kirk Wallace as cited in Health Canada 2000)

TO the Patient is a Nonexistent to Low Level of Engagement

At this level (level 1), the patient is mostly involved or informed rather than engaged. Information is delivered *TO* the individual patient and family via fact sheets, patient-care guides, or advertisements, such as the pharmaceutical commercials that flood us with a lot of information in a very short amount of time. This level of involvement with PFACs and other patient groups only notifies and explains processes or programs that are already in place, where decisions have already been made. At this level of passive engagement, or really involvement, the patient voice is nonexistent and does not have any influence on decisions, policies, or outcomes.

Systems that listen *TO* the patient begin to move from involvement to a low level of engagement:

At this level (level 2), health care systems and providers gather information from individual patients and families by asking passive questions about their symptoms and/or concerns, "What's bothering you?" At this level, information is gathered from larger groups of patients and families via public comment opportunities, focus groups, questionnaires, and surveys. The patient voice is present at this level, but it does not necessarily influence decisions, policies, or outcomes.

FOR the Patient is a More Moderate Level of Engagement

This level (level 3) encourages discussion *FOR* the benefit of patients and families, where health systems and providers have a mutual interest in an issue that may or may not lead to a mutually beneficial solution. At this level, individual patients may be encouraged to have a discussion about their symptoms, and/or concerns, with the use of more active questions, "What can we do for you?" Larger groups of patients can participate in advisory councils, advisory boards, and round table discussions that focus on what they can do *FOR* patients and families. The patient and family voice begins to be more integrated into what can be done *FOR* the patient, and can be passive or active. The voice at this level may or may not have influence on decisions, policies, or outcomes.

WITH the Patient Begins a Higher Level of Engagement

At this level (level 4), health systems and providers engage *WITH* individual patients and families to set goals and make shared decisions. At this level, larger groups of patients and families can be seen in work groups and committees, where mutually beneficial goals are worked on *WITH* patients, but which goals to work on are not necessarily decided by patients. The patient and family voice is actively present, and it will likely have an influence on decisions, policies, and outcomes.

Partnering *WITH* patients to develop solutions is at the highest level of engagement:

At this level (level 5), goals are conceptualized together, and set out to achieve a mutually beneficial solution through collaboration. The system and patients work side by side, co-designing plans, and even co-investigating research. The health system and patients agree on best ways to implement plans into practice. The voice is most active and influential at this level, where success depends on collaboration and partnership.

Successful examples of patient collaboration can be found in numerous partnerships between patients and hospitals. A PFAC member, and patient, mentioned during a meeting how much better it is to heal when it's quiet—noting that the in-patient areas of the hospital are noisy places where patients cannot rest at night. The PFAC worked with the hospital to come up with a set of best practices to quiet the patient areas at night. Not only did the new practices lead to an increase in patient satisfaction, other hospitals took note and followed suit. At a pediatric hospital, the parents of the PFAC noted that the children who were having teeth surgically removed in the outpatient dental unit were sad when returning home without a tooth to put under the pillow for the tooth fairy. The PFAC worked with child life representatives of the hospital to provide small surprise gifts from the "tooth fairy" left for the children in the recovery room.

Emplace plans into practice. Sometimes even the best laid out plans seem to fall wayside for lack of follow through. Such as "weren't we going to start..." and "oh yeah, we never let so and so know..." Other times, plans cannot be implemented for a number of reasons, and that's ok, but it is not simply enough to ask for patient feedback and input. You need to circle back, and let folks know what changes are being worked on and how they will be put into practice, as well as when plans cannot be implemented and why. If you are going to encourage and welcome the patient voice, you need to close the loop on the engagement cycle.

Communication is key. Think about the last time you asked a friend or family member for help or their advice. They may have helped you with an important decision or helped lay out a plan to tackle a problem. Whether you chose to listen to their advice or follow through with the plan or not, one thing is almost certain. The next time you spoke with them they likely asked how things panned out. You were likely eager to follow up with them, and thanked them for their assistance. Your friend was probably happy to be informed and felt valued; and the next time you need help, they will likely be happy to assist. It's human nature to be curious about a turn of events, but, more importantly, people need to feel valued for their opinion and thanked for their efforts. The same is true when engaging with patients and families. Even the highest level of engagement depends on communication and follow-up. When patients are engaged in a plan or project, and given an opportunity to contribute their voice, they feel valued. However if they never hear back on how their voice may have helped influence change, the value gets lost and they are less likely to use their voice the next time it's needed.

If we look back at the public involvement continuum from Health Canada again, we see that true engagement does not move on a spectrum from left to right only, it goes back from right to left again. Authentic engagement moves from informing, to listening, to consulting, to partnering, but partnering successfully is contingent on

Fig. 1.2 Circle of engagement. (© Alexis Snyder, 2018)

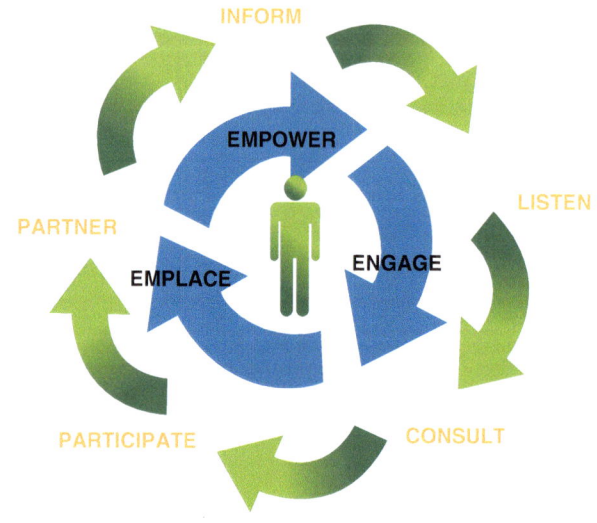

consulting, listening, and sending information back again. So, perhaps, another way to look at this continuum of engagement is not from left to right and back again, but as a continuous circle of events, all connected to the 3 E's: Empower, Engage, and Emplace (Fig. 1.2).

Common Obstacles to Patient Engagement

Understanding how to best engage with and hear the patient voice is only the beginning. To truly have the patient voice represented across all aspects of the health care system, the obstacles that prevent it from happening need to be understood. Even when providers and health systems have the skills and tools in place to achieve authentic engagement, the patient voice may still be difficult to hear, or altogether muted.

One of the first and, sometimes, most prominent stumbling blocks is poor communication. As touched upon earlier, a provider may have communication skills and a wonderful rapport with their patient, but the channels to foster that communication may be in need of repair.

Take, for instance, Mary.[1] Mary is experiencing gastrointestinal (GI) pain and is referred by her GI provider to a sub-specialist and instructed to call and make an appointment. The next day, Mary calls the specialist's office and is informed by the scheduler that patients are not allowed to switch physicians and she will not book the appointment. Mary tries to explain that she was instructed to call, but her voice goes unheard. Mary reaches back out to the first specialist, and has a difficult time getting in touch with them, leaves messages with their scheduler, and so on and so forth. For days nothing gets done about scheduling the appointment;

Mary's voice is lost in the system. Mary, who is at the center, is actually stuck in the middle and her pain is getting worse. Eventually, weeks later, she is finally able to speak with the first specialist. They are shocked to learn that she was unable to book an appointment on her own, and the provider now steps in to help get the appointment scheduled. When Mary finally sees the sub-specialist, they too are shocked to learn that she had such difficulty scheduling and was told that she was not allowed to "switch" physicians. This is a clear example of a lack of communication, and the channels in place to help coordinate services for the patient created stress for the patient, prolonged pain, and caused a longer than necessary wait time to receive care. How could this experience have been more patient-centered? Communication is key between all the players involved. The patient's voice would have been better received when making the phone call if the first provider's office had spoken with the sub-specialist office before the patient called. Once Mary was feeling better, she was able to share this story with hospital administrators and engage in solutions with the provider's office. This is a prime example of why the patient voice is so important in process improvement. Without the patient voice at the system level, more patients would continue to encounter this mishap, which is more than just frustrating—the delay in making the appointment can lead to poor health outcomes.

Another often overlooked area of communication that creates a barrier to engagement is low health literacy skills, which is often confused with low literacy. Literacy, commonly known as "the ability to read and write" and expanded to mean "understand, communicate and gain useful knowledge [18]," is not the same thing as health literacy. A person can have the highest degree of education and high literacy skills to function in society, but not be fluent in medical terminology or how the health system works. Health literacy depends on the lay people's knowledge of health topics and affects the individual's ability to navigate the health care system [19]. According to the National Action Plan to Improve Health, nine out of ten adults lack proficient health literacy skills [20].

Without strong skills in health literacy, it can be very difficult for a patient to find their way through the ever-changing sea of health care. Trying to stay afloat in a world where medical jargon and technical terms sound like a foreign language is almost impossible, and certainly taxing. Even when a patient may have proficient health literacy, the anxiety and/or physical distress over an illness can impact the way they process important information about their health. Patients may not understand medical guidelines, which may lead to poor health outcomes. If a patient is unable to understand their diagnosis and/or the information received, how can they engage?

So how do we solve the problem of health literacy and its blockades to patient-centeredness and engagement? Well, that's a loaded question which could take up a chapter or an entire book on its own. But some simple places to start with individual patients and families are to provide information in lay terms and in ways that take into account the individual needs of the patient or family member. Such as simple and easy verbal, as well as written, instructions without medical jargon, drawing pictures or diagrams, or even demonstrating a health-related task, such as an injection. It is also helpful to explain why this treatment or action is important, and the expected impact it will have on their condition.

Empower patients to use their voice to ask questions, as well as to inform providers if and when they don't understand. Remember that it can be very intimidating to be a patient, who is sometimes sitting vulnerably in a paper gown, while a clinician in a suit and/or white coat stands over them. When possible, give information and instructions on a level playing field, by giving the patient the opportunity to get dressed and sit down to discuss their health and treatment options. Consider that even though a patient may acknowledge what you are saying by nodding their head, they still may not understand.

Practice active engagement and ask the patient to repeat back what they understand, explaining that you want to be certain you are explaining in a way they can receive and remember it. Take time to consider the cultural differences that might also be at play, not just language barriers. When working with groups of patients, such as in an advisory council, it is also important to speak in terms that everyone in the room can understand—no abbreviations, medical terminology, or jargon that may convey the feeling of a secret language and, possibly, inferiority.

Cultural competence, which can be described as the health systems' or providers' ability to take into account the cultural beliefs, values, and preferences of diverse populations, also plays a role. Take,[1] for example, the story of a young mother whose child had a long-term hospital admission. During their stay, the mother was routinely approached by nurses, physicians, and other support staff to engage in conversation and decision-making about her child's care. The mother was reluctant to engage in conversation and deferred the conversation until her husband arrived later in the evening. On several occasions, the staff also invited the mother to attend social support groups with the other parents, where lunch was served. When staff would approach with the invitation she would politely nod and avoid eye contact. She would occasionally attend, but did not eat. The staff could not understand why she would not engage with them, make eye contact, or eat during these events. Assuming she might like to eat in private, they would often re-heat her a plate and bring it to her later in the day. She still never ate it, so eventually the staff stopped bringing it.

The mother began to feel that the staff was ambivalent toward her, she couldn't figure out why, and eventually she stopped attending the support groups, and stopped engaging with the staff altogether. Later, she would tell her husband that she felt the staff did not like her because she was not American, and the family requested to transfer their child to another hospital, a move that might have been detrimental to the child's health. The staff were dumbfounded to hear this, feeling as though they had made every effort to make this family feel comfortable and supported.

What the staff did not know is that this mother's culture was different from theirs. In her culture, women do not look men or other authority figures directly in the eye and they do not make any decisions for the family, as the patriarch of the family does. She was not trying to be disrespectful but quite the contrary. As for not eating what was offered to her? Her religion did not allow her to eat the foods being offered. If the staff had taken the time to engage in a different way with this mother and learn about her family's individual values, a number of misconceptions may have been avoided, the information needed to help care for the patient and support the family could have been gained quicker, and the request to make a risky transfer could have been avoided. And while it may have seemed to the staff that this mother was not willing to engage, she just needed to be approached in a different manner and empowered to use her voice in the best way she could when considering her personal values and beliefs.

Time can also be an issue for providers and patients and health systems. Providers may struggle with a busy schedule and lack of time to fully engage a patient during an appointment, or communicate in between visits. Setting aside enough time ahead of schedule to fully engage with a patient 1:1 can have system-wide restraints that can't be resolved in this chapter. What can be emphasized is, if falling behind schedule, don't rush. Each patient deserves equal time, and needs it. I never mind waiting for a provider if I know that, when it's my turn, I will receive the same time and respect as the patient before me.

Patients may also struggle with finding time to attend meetings. Make every effort to provide a variety of ways for patients to actively participate. Meeting every month at 10 am because the space at the hospital is available then may not work for everyone. For example if the patient works full time from 9 to 5, perhaps offering a meeting time every other month in the evening, or offering meetings during the lunch hour would allow them an opportunity to attend. Consider adding phone or web conferencing for those who may be available but can't be there in person. Outreach to invite patients into the conversation is often lacking. A health system can't expect to have patients and families engage in system activities, such as an advisory council, if they do not make the activities widely known and advertised.

Health systems may struggle with finding time to schedule advisory council meetings or other committee or board meetings, where the patient voice needs to be heard. Planning time to engage with patients and families is a necessity. Systems can't expect to deliver patient-centered care that does not involve the patient voice, so they need to take time to engage patients and families if they truly want to be patient-centered, or provide care that is respectful and responsive to individual preferences and needs. Consider for a moment buying a new car. You're now probably thinking "Buying a car?" and "What the heck does that have to do with health care?"

Patients are consumers of the health care system, whose needs can only be identified if they are given the opportunity to voice them. Medicine is not one size fits all. Neither are cars. Let's say you are a family of four with a dog, you travel by car often with lots of luggage, a car seat, and a stroller. Now let's say you call a car dealership and state your need of a new vehicle. You have no further voice in what kind of car you would like, or what is important to you. The dealer simply sends over a 2-passenger smart car. Does this car meet your needs? Are you satisfied with it? Probably not. You call the dealer and try to voice that this car doesn't work for you, but they can't understand it because their other customers love it and the logo for the smart car says "Not too big, Not too small, Just Right [21]." But just right for whom? It certainly isn't right for your family of four, your dog, and your luggage. This is exactly what can happen in medicine if the patients and families who are at the receiving end of services do not have a voice in what works for whom, when, and under what circumstances.

Another hardship to engaging with patients and families is fear of the unknown. Providers and health systems can be fearful of hearing complaints. In any valued relationship, an open and honest dialog is important. Hearing dissatisfaction, in a constructive way, is the first step to improvement. By nature, we all tend to protect ourselves and our self-esteem by avoiding feedback we feel is negative, or a threat to our sense of self or well-being. Feedback, however, does not have to be negative and, when engaging with patients, if you take a step back, listen, and work together on a solution, it will benefit everyone in the end.

There are many obstacles to overcome when engaging with patients and families, and while these are only a few examples, it is imperative that health care systems explore the obstacles within their own environment and commit to practices that ensure that the patient and family voice is always present and well represented, whether it be 1:1, or in the larger world of patient advisory.

A Seat at the Table

Understanding the value of the patient and caregiver voice, it's time to think about securing a place at the table for them. While many hospitals and health systems may utilize a PFAC to incorporate the patient voice into service delivery, patients and families are still underrepresented on other boards and committees. Their voice needs to be upfront and present in all aspects of system improvement, such as on quality and safety committees. However, leadership is sometimes reluctant to have the patient in the room for fear of the patient hearing too much. They may worry that the patient will be privy to events that may reflect poorly on the system and in some way be retaliated on. This thought process couldn't be more wrong and, besides, the patient who has lived experience within the health care system has likely already experienced similar issues and captivating the patient perspective on why things may have gone astray, as well as what could have happened differently, is an important piece of making it work for the next patient.

Health systems need to be transparent, build relationships with patient and families, and welcome the patient into the room. Patients aren't waking in the morning and trying to figure out a way that they can become a health care spy and take an organization down. Quite the contrary, they are waking with a voice in their head that says, "How can I make a difference?" not only in services that affect the care and treatment received by them or their loved ones but for patients everywhere.

Leadership must welcome these eyes, ears, and voices, and be committed to engaging and partnering with patients. Their lived experience can shine a new light on the work being done. I can't count the number of times I have sat in a room full of clinicians, administrators, insurers, and/or researchers and heard, "I never would have thought about it that way" and "that changes everything."

Patients need a seat at the table throughout the multiple channels of health care delivery. Today, patients have seats on steering committees, advisory boards, roundtables, hearings, ethics panels, IRBs (Internal Review Boards) and much more. So where are some of the seats at the table being reserved? The FDA (The Food and Drug Administration), CMS (Centers for Medicare and Medicaid Services), the AAP (American Academy of Pediatrics) are just a few places that are incorporating patients into planning. The Yale Center for Outcomes Research and Evaluation Services (CORE) and the Patient Centered Outcomes Research Institute (PCORI) are incorporating the patient and family voice in patient-centered outcomes research. More and more professional conferences on patient-centered care, and other patient-related topics, are inviting patients in to partake in the information process, but also to engage as speakers, panel members, workshop presenters, and as members of the planning committees. Some hospitals even include patients as part of the interviewing process for new staff, and in patient rounding. And let's not forget that a patient and caregiver is writing this chapter and is part of the editorial team.

While patients as advisors are starting to spread into these areas, their voices are still largely underrepresented and lack in diversity. It is not enough to start a patient advisory council, or open the boardroom doors to include patients and families at the table. Patient-centered medicine is not cookie cutter, and, therefore, health systems must bring patients from diverse backgrounds, cultures, ages, and skills to the table.

Let's say you are in need of knee surgery, but you are unsure of your options and need to consult with a surgeon. You book an appointment and show up at the hospital. It's your lucky day. You are told you will be seeing three physicians to give you a range of perspectives. Wow, you feel like you just won the lottery! You take a seat at the table with the physicians. One by one they introduce themselves: a gynecologist, a dentist, and a pediatrician (and no, there is not a joke coming about the three doctors that walk into the bar…) Will any of these physicians, no matter how skilled at what they do, be able to give you the perspective and information you need to make an informed choice? Of course not.

The same is true when consulting and partnering with patients. It is not enough to just bring patients into the equation. Health systems must work with diverse populations of patients and families and afford opportunities for varied patient voices, with varied experiences, from varied backgrounds to be available to advise and work on a given topic. After all, if a system is looking to engage with patients on a project to improve outcomes, let's say for children from low socio-economic status with poor access to dental care, they are not going to get too much help if they partner with patients of higher socio-economic status, without children, and/or who have easy access to dental services.

Patient Engagement in Research

Never has there been a more exciting time in history of medical research. Research that once only focused on clinical outcomes has begun a new movement known as Patient-Centered Outcomes Research, or PCOR. In 2010, with legislation from the Patient Protection and Affordable Care Act [22], congress authorized the creation of The Patient Centered Outcomes Research Institute (PCORI) in Washington, D.C. They tasked them with a mandate to close the gap on decisional dilemmas for patients and providers, by answering questions not usually addressed by traditional research methods, and thus PCOR began [23]. What exactly is PCOR? According to PCORI, "PCOR helps people and their caregivers communicate and make informed health care decisions, allowing their voices to be heard in assessing the value of health care options" and "answers patient-centered questions, such as:

Given my personal characteristics, conditions, and preferences, what should I expect will happen to me?

What are my options, and what are the potential benefits and harms of those options?

What can I do to improve the outcomes that are most important to me?

How can clinicians and the care delivery systems they work in help me make the best decisions about my health and health care?" [24]

Answering questions like these are patient-centeredness at its best, and can make a real difference in decision making for patients, as well as their providers. But is there a place for the patient voice in the research process itself? You bet there is. Patients can and should be engaged in the research process upfront and throughout the research cycle. And with the work being done at PCORI, they are. Unlike traditional models of research, the projects funded by PCORI require patients, caregivers, and other stakeholders to actively participate in the research, not as subjects, but as partners. Patients help identify the outcomes of importance, help form research questions and aims, can be involved in data collection and analysis, and are expected to be an integral part of the dissemination process.

Authentically engaging patients in research makes the results more relevant. Understanding what matters most to patients at the start of the research ensures getting it right the first time and produces results that really matter to patients and caregivers. One such study funded by PCORI looked at nonsurgical methods for aortic value replacement. The principal investigator's (PI) outcome goals were to determine which technique would provide the best chance of survival. However, when the PI sat down with a group of older patients partnering in the study, they voiced their primary concern and fear was not of death, but of adverse events, such as stroke, that might leave them dependent on someone else's care at home or in a nursing facility. By working with patients, the PI was able to determine what mattered most to the patient, and he updated the outcome measures to include discharge to home or nursing facility. Ultimately, the study found that a non-surgical method to replace the aortic value to be as safe as surgery and allowed more patients to go home from the hospital rather than to a nursing facility [25].

Patients and caregivers are also being engaged in the funding review processes of organizations, such as PCORI, and governmental agencies, such as

HRSA (Health Resource and Services Administration) and the Department of Defense, to ensure evaluation of the patient-centered aspects of the study. And, as many PCOR funded studies are coming to fruition, patients are also engaged as peer reviewers and in reviewing projects up for dissemination and implementation awards.

Next Steps/Hopes for the Future

We have come a long way since the days of, "My doctor knows best and they will make the right decision for me." Patients are more often being encouraged to engage in their own health care. Patients are becoming an integral part of the planning, development, and implementation and evaluation of policies and programs that affect the care and services delivered to the broader population of patients and families. Patients have lived experience with the systems of care available to them. Their voice is unique. It needs not only to be heard but to be partnered with to improve the quality of care and services we all receive, some more than others. And while we may have come a long way, we still have a long way to go.

My own voice, that of a patient, caregiver, and advocate, has shared some information on the importance of the patient voice, but it is only that of one. My hope is that if you are a patient reading this, you feel empowered to engage in your own health care and the larger systems of care that affects others. Never be afraid to speak up and use your voice. Words are powerful, and your engagement and partnership can lead to change. Never feel like you can't ask questions or offer solutions. Keep calm and collaborate.

If you are a provider, system administrator, or other health services leader, I hope you are empowered to empower, engage, and partner with patients and families, embrace their voices, and emplace plans into practices. And remember, if you are going to ask for patient input, be open, fully listen and be prepared to change. Don't be fearful of the patient voice. You are the experts of medicine; patients are the experts of living with their bodies and health conditions, and you need to work together.

I leave you with a powerful thought on the patient voice and caregiver voice. A voice patients and caregivers were able to use out of a collaboration with researchers, and providers, when engaged as partners in a research project to uncover the challenges and obstacles to coordinating care for children with complex medical conditions. A voice they previously described as "often muted by judgement or lack of understanding" that can be improved with "open and honest communication without egos [26]."

The patient voice may be a difficult instrument to play, but it is far more difficult when once learned there is no one there to hear it.

Acknowledgement Thank you to my dear friend and colleague, Dr. Pranavi V. Sreeramoju, for empowering me by inviting me to engage in this book project; and for Springer Publishing and the rest of the editorial team for emplacing my voice through words into the hands of others. And most of all, to Sara. Without you, I would not be the mother, caregiver, advocate, and better person that I am today. I love you to the moon and back.

References

1. https://www.brainyquote.com/topics/human_voice. Retrieved on May 16, 2018.
2. Committee on Quality Health Care in America, Institute of Medicine. Crossing the quality chasm: a new health system for the 21st century. Washington, DC: National Academy Press; 2001.
3. Charmenl PA, Frampton SB. Building the business case for patient-centered care. Healthc Financ Manage. 2008;62(3):80–5.
4. Stewart M, et al. The impact of patient-centered care on outcomes. J Fam Pract. 2000;49(9):796–804.
5. http://www.dana-farber.org/for-patients-and-families/becoming-a-patient/patient-safety-and-advocacy/patient-and-family-advisory-councils/adult-patient-and-family-advisory-council/. Retrieved on May 7, 2018.
6. Wieczorek CC, Nowak P, Frampton SB, Pelikan JM. Strengthening patient and family engagement in healthcare – The New Haven Recommendations. Patient Educ Couns. 2018;101(8):1508–13.
7. https://www.hcfama.org/patient-and-family-advisory-councils-pfacs. Retrieved on May 7, 2018.
8. Patient Family Advisory Councils, Mass. Dept. of Public Health Circular Letter: DHCQ 09-07-514. Mass.gov retrieved on April 26, 2020.
9. Health Care for All. 2015 annual assessment of Massachusetts patient and family advisory councils. Dec 2015. HCFAMA.org. Retrieved on May 7, 2018.
10. The Beryl Institute. Defining patient experience. http://www.theberylinstitute.org/?page=DefiningPatientExp. Retrieved on May 10, 2014.
11. Carmen KL, Dardess P, Maurer M, et al. Patient and family engagement: a framework for understanding the elements and developing interventions and policies. Health Aff (Millwood). 2013;32:223–31.
12. CMS. HCAHPS: patients' perspectives of care survey. CMS.Gov. Retrieved on May 14, 2018.
13. Mayo Clinic. Convergence insufficiency. Patient Care and Health Information-Diseases and Conditions. July 15, 2017. http://www.Mayoclinic.org. Retrieved on May 25, 2018.
14. Hospitality. Dictionary.com unabridged. n.d. Retrieved May 6, 2018 from Dictionary.com website http://www.dictionary.com/browse/hospitality.
15. Macleod D. Engagement vs. involvement. Feb 19, 2012. http://www.thoughtexchange.com. Retrieved on May 16, 2018.
16. Health Canada. From Wikipedia, the free encyclopedia. http://www.en.wikipedia.org. Retrieved on May 16, 2018.
17. https://www.canada.ca/en/health-canada/corporate/about-health-canada/reports-publications/health-canada-policy-toolkit-public-involvement-decision-making.html#a1. Retried May 22, 2018.
18. http://www.en.m.wikipedia.org. Literacy. Retrieved on May 22, 2018.
19. http://www.health.gov. Quick guide to Health Literacy fact sheet. Retrieved on May 22, 2018.
20. U.S. Department of Health and Human Services, Office of Disease Prevention and Health Promotion. National action plan to improve health literacy. Washington, DC: Author; 2010.
21. https://www.smartusa.com. Retrieved on May 22, 2018.
22. Patient Protection and Affordable Care Act, 42 U.S.C. § 18001. 2010.
23. Patient-Centered Outcomes Research Institute, 2012 Annual Report. p. 2.
24. https://www.pcoi.org/research&results/patinetcenteredoutcomesresearch. Retrieved May 24, 2018.
25. PCORI. A less invasive way to replace a heart value: is newer better? Feb 22, 2018. Pcori.org. Research and results retrieved on May 25, 2018.
26. Carosella A, Snyder A, Ward E. What parents of children with complex medical conditions want their child's physicians to understand. JAMA Pediatr. 2018;172(4):315–6. https://doi.org/10.1001/jamapediatrics.2017.3931.

Voice of the Physician

2

Stephen G. Weber

Introduction

To fully understand the perspective of physicians on issues of quality, safety, value and patient-centered care, one needs to appreciate the context in which doctors have been engaged in the multitude of changes that have come to medical practice in the United States over the past 20 years. As has already been observed, too often, doctors have felt that changes have been done *to* them, not *for* them and certainly never *with* them. Moreover, as recently pointed out in a *New York Times* editorial circulated widely in physician lounges (where such places still exist!), physicians have been asked or even expected to shoulder without assistance the burden of an increasingly demanding health care environment, while investments and resources are showered on technology, administrators and consultants [1].

That the industry is out of balance is supported by the phenomenon that has followed the quality and safety movement as the next great issue in American health care. Physician burnout and the erosion of resilience in the profession are described as an epidemic. The cost of this epidemic is measured in talented colleagues leaving the profession and promising young people electing to fulfill their potential in other more lucrative and less demanding fields. More alarming is the recognition of the increased risk for self-destructive behavior and even suicide among physicians in the United States. Coming full circle, there is increasing evidence that patients also pay a dire price for physician burnout, with increased harm events, poor outcomes and dissatisfaction with care [2].

From a broader view, serious questions remain whether the widely-endorsed commitment to patient-centered clinical care, quality and access is even working. The so-called cost curve for American medicine is not reliably bending

S. G. Weber (✉)
The University of Chicago Medicine, Chicago, IL, USA
e-mail: sgweber@medicine.bsd.uchicago.edu

© Springer Nature Switzerland AG 2020
P. V. Sreeramoju et al. (eds.), *The Patient and Health Care System: Perspectives on High-Quality Care*, https://doi.org/10.1007/978-3-030-46567-4_2

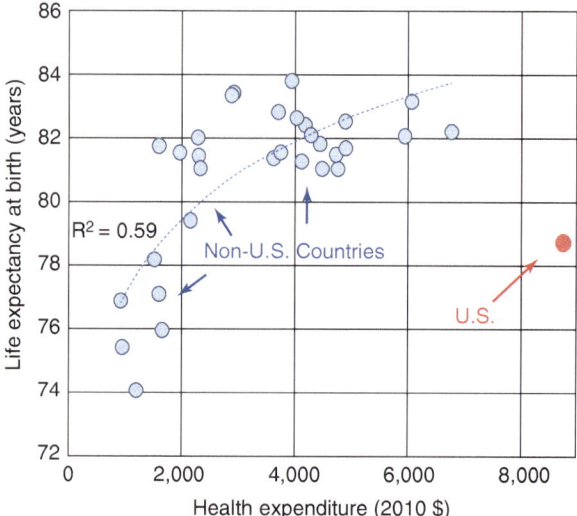

Fig. 2.1 Value in health (US vs. international comparisons). The chart demonstrates health care expenditures to life expectancy at birth for the United States vs. 32 international comparators. (Source: Data are from World Bank – World Development Indicators (http://data.worldbank.org/data-catalog/world-development-indicators) and OECD (https://stats.oecd.org/) via Esteban Ortiz-Ospina and Max Roser (2018) – "Financing Health Care". https://ourworldindata.org/financing-healthcare with a Creative Commons CC BY-SA 3.0 AU license)

under the weight of incentives, restructuring and transparency. Critics and supporters alike of the Affordable Care Act acknowledge the limitations of the massive legislative intervention. Despite the attention and investment, American patients have not yet enjoyed improvements in meaningful clinical outcomes when compared with similar nations around the globe (Fig. 2.1). Could it be that we are discovering just how little the health system and care delivery in the United States can be improved *without* fully engaging and supporting our most important resource: physicians?

That is not to say that physicians have not been involved. A large number of physicians have crossed the administrative, if not the quality, chasm in order to assume leadership roles in quality, safety and patient experience. Leaders, and even superstars, have emerged, notably expanding the disciplines of implementation and health care delivery science. However, for the larger majority, the struggle remains for physicians who are deeply committed to the work in quality and safety. In academic centers, the roles are rarely endorsed as a basis for academic promotion or recognition. In the community, the physician who takes on volunteer (or even modestly paid) work in this space must surrender the lost revenue of not seeing patients or doing procedures.

Apart from these groups, what remains are the many thousands of talented and dedicated physicians who are committed to patient care and follow the calling that brought them to the field in the first place. For these individuals, there is no intention to "buy down time" or to publish in top-notch journals. Rather, they only want the opportunity to do what is best for their patients, while *enjoying* a fulfilling and productive professional career. This chapter is intended to focus on these individuals.

Over the next pages, we will examine some of the major trends in health care over the past several years. Each is aimed to embrace and enhance the themes of patient-centeredness and improved outcomes. At the same time, and perhaps unsurprisingly, in lived experience, each has emerged as a potential driver of physician disengagement. We will briefly review each of these trends and how we got to this point. Then we will turn and offer a different perspective of what it could look like going forward if the perspective and values of physicians are aligned for success in each case. The chapter ends with advice to patients about how they can make a difference and what they might expect in terms of the role of their own physician in improving outcomes and driving change. Because in the end, even where we highlight the significance and importance of the physicians or any caregivers, the patient should and must always remain at the center and lead the care team.

Interdisciplinary Care

The role and number of non-physician providers in clinical care has expanded dramatically in the past 30 years. Physician assistants, advanced practice nurses, clinical pharmacists, to name just a few, have increasingly been promoted and deployed as essential members of the modern care team. Much of this has been driven by need. As care has become more complex and the needs of patients have evolved, demand for access has increased and the expectation on providers to approach patients more holistically has broadened, compelling the inclusion of individuals trained with various and sometimes complementary skill sets.

For patients, advanced practice professionals can be a godsend, especially once expectations are set and managed. While some are occasionally riled at the prospect of not seeing a physician for even the most mundane complaint, increasingly they are developing close and warm bonds of trust and confidence in the non-physicians involved in their care. Such patients enjoy the benefits of improved access, enhanced communication and potentially improved outcomes with respect to both clinical care and utilization.

Supplementing the professional team over the past decade or more has been an equally substantial expansion in the role of additional specialists to support specific activities and outcomes. Practices and programs aligned towards population health and risk-based contracting are adding care navigators, coaches and community health workers to their care teams. Financial counselors, behavioral health social workers and a host of coordinators frequently round out the group.

And while these investments, if deployed wisely, should enhance the collective effectiveness of the care team to the benefit of patients, new problems have emerged. Advanced practice providers, owing to a combination of inconsistent licensing regulations across jurisdictions, institutional history and culture, as well as resentment by some physicians, are too frequently compelled to work below their actual scope of practice. In some settings, imprecision in compensation and incentive models turn physicians and advanced practice providers into potential rivals, competing for the same patients and productivity credits. Other team members are sometimes not fully or consistently engaged in practice, poorly understood by some members of the care team and therefore deployed irregularly and not to maximal effect. To the patient, care is perceived as fragmented and poor communication between team members creates not only dissatisfaction but increases the risk for poor outcomes and even harm events.

The finely tuned care team of the future need not suffer these shortcomings. Team care is not going away and, in fact, must become the norm, in order to deliver the outcomes, access, experience and affordability at the center of value-based care. That is not to say that these teams will be uniform, a single model deployed homogenously across all populations and practices. Rather, the care team of the future is specifically designed around the patients being served. In this approach, the physiologic, pharmacologic, psychological, social, economic and spiritual needs of a patient are identified and validated. Experienced clinicians, together with administrators and other stakeholders, take time to consider this inventory when making investments in personnel and skill sets. In every case, clinicians are given responsibility for only those needs for which they are uniquely qualified to deliver. By engaging in this process, physicians and other team members are not only aware of, but invested in, the value of the truly multidisciplinary team.

Having articulated the responsibilities of each team member, individual and role accountability must be carefully aligned with incentives and compensation. Ideally, team members share goals linked to that which is valued by patients: outcomes, experience, access and cost. In each domain, team members have line of sight to their contribution to those outcomes, as measured in specific processes and expectations that they must fulfill. Role descriptions and expected activities should be reviewed together with the entire team to avoid both redundancy and missed opportunities for shared success. When in action in service of patients, the care team must place a premium on communication. Successful teams begin and end each session of work with huddles in which transparency and candor are essential. Team training, akin to that which is practiced in other industries yields benefit in building trust, confidence and effectiveness.

This deliberate approach will not immediately undo the cultural and historical challenges that come with new and blended roles and expertise. We practice now in an environment in which newer advanced practice professions are challenging the status quo of physician leadership at a time when physicians already feel threatened by a loss of autonomy and fulfillment. Time alone will likely prove to be the greatest salve as successive generations of interdisciplinary teams enter training and practice together. However, close professional practice on optimized teams should accelerate this process.

The Electronic Medical Record

One of the most talked about changes in care delivery over the past 30 years has been the proliferation of the electronic medical record (EMR) and its interposition between patients and clinicians in practice. Spurred by generous financial incentives and elaborate expectations, the EMR was promoted and ultimately sold on the promise of interoperability. In the digital future, American patients would benefit from unprecedented portability to move through a complex system to meet their individual needs for health and wellness. Unencumbered by the tyranny of having received care in one or another place, quality-seeking health care consumers would unleash the free market to drive competition and improvement to the benefit of all. The idealized EMR would drive enormous gains in safety, quality and satisfaction.

The lived reality has of course been quite different and often distressing. Physicians routinely decry the EMR as the bane of their clinical existence, and the narrative of senior physicians driven to early retirement abounds. Even the younger so-called digital natives are incensed – frustrated that the EMR lacks the easy functionality and user interfaces with which they routinely book travel, stream movies and music and make online purchases. The EMR has been broadly implicated in the epidemic of burnout as physicians struggle to unplug from work during off hours, bound not only by the proliferation of clinical documentation, but an array of seemingly new regulatory and billing requirements. Patients complain that the ubiquitous laptops, tablets and workstations literally are coming between them and their doctors. Finally, the promise of easy interoperability and improved safety: unfulfilled at best and worsened in many cases.

One cannot argue that the perspective of physicians was entirely excluded from the original intrusion of the EMR into American health care. Physicians in practice in the 1990s and later can attest to invaluable hours committed away from patient care to participate in focus groups, portfolio committees and user-acceptance testing. Closer to the inevitable "go-live" physicians huddled in classrooms or endured endless computer-based training modules to ensure we could maximize the bells and whistles of the new systems. But was this degree of engagement authentic and were the values, dedication and experience of physicians really applied to version 1.0 of the EMR in the United States.? How could things have been done differently and what can be done moving forward to upgrade the system?

The next generation of electronic health records will surely benefit from more meaningful and expert leadership by physicians. The burgeoning field of medical informatics, now a board-certified sub-specialty unto itself, is formalizing and recognizing the training and expertise of physicians committed to the interface between clinical care and technology. With the democratization of this knowledge and focus to a broader and more diverse class of physician leaders, standards of evidence and practice are being developed and deployed as in any clinical practice.

The leadership of this group will undoubtedly focus on advancing towards the unfulfilled aspiration of interoperability, for in this alone comes the greatest dividend of the electronic record. Meaningful incentives from payers (including the federal government) will compel standards for data and file sharing that will spur the innovation to resolve even the most vexing challenges of system compatibility and cyber security. Even as the landscape supports greater corporate diversification (for almost no vital industry exists with only two main competitors), physicians on the frontlines will embrace a general move away from customization in accordance with prior practice in favor of standards driven by usability and efficiency.

At this more human level, additional changes abound. Applying rational and evidence-based approaches to learning theory, physicians and other clinicians will be provided with customized and ongoing training and education at the point of care to enhance the effective use of the electronic health record. Those who oversee an increasingly employed and salaried physician workforce will make investments in both analytics to identify needs as well as unique and novel educational programming to ensure that physicians remain efficient but also satisfied, for the cost of turnover for a physician or surgeon is enormous.

At the intersection of medical informatics and implementation science, physician investigators and innovators will introduce new technology and practices that lower the technological barrier between patients and physicians, allowing for a less obtrusive and impersonal interface with technology in the exam room. High fidelity voice recognition will allow for not only accurate documentation of the encounter but will also facilitate the implementation of care plans, communication between team members and education of the patient to better engage them in their own care.

In some respects, patients and physicians today find themselves at the nadir of experience with the EMR. Digital capabilities outpaced the readiness of our profession to meaningfully shape the touch, feel and effectiveness of the new technology. Physicians expected less experienced and less expert observers to mimic contemporary practice in a digital space without fully understanding the consequences of this suboptimal approach. Going forward, physicians at the nexus of clinical practice and technology, ever mindful of the needs of the patients they serve, will be in the lead, helping us to understand how the technology can be used to leverage improved practice and outcomes, while supporting both the clinical team and those who entrust us with their care.

(Big) Data

Whenever a group of health system or payer leaders, health care commentators or consultants gather, at least one will eventually invoke the importance of "big data." Imprecisely defined around advanced analytics, predictive algorithms and techniques, big data promises to bring to health care the improvements in service delivery, finances and personalization enjoyed by a multitude of other industries. What physician or hospital leader has not been pitched on the merits of the next Lyft, Yelp or Alexa for health care?

The superficial appeal of big data is not only attractive but also seems rational and aligned with clinicians trained and experienced in principles to evidence-based care. Amplified and accelerated by the promise of the EMR, data are now available that describe the clinical history, experience, exposures, management, treatment and response of individual patients under care. Paired with interoperability between systems and sites of care, what emerges is a flawed, but more holistic digital representation of every patient. Such data and perspectives can and should then be plumbed by sophisticated analytic models to extract actionable information to optimize care.

Early adopters in the application of big data in medicine include cancer investigators and clinicians who have captured essential and complicated genetic information about both tumors and patients in order to help guide treatment. These therapies themselves are informed by advanced analytics and modeling, from the design of novel therapeutics to deterministic models that predict the best and customized course of therapy. "Personalized" cancer care has become the norm in both the clinical literature and in patient-facing advertisement and promotion. The approach is now spreading to other domains and specialties, meeting a consumer-driven appetite for individualized care.

The quality and safety movement has likewise been attracted to and driven by progressively bigger and bigger data. The early days of single-institution observational reports regarding risk factors, prediction models and outcome analyses have given way to more sophisticated and meaningful approaches. Cluster randomized trials examine the impact of infection prevention strategies across networks of acute care hospitals. Confusing, confounding factors and covariates are managed more effectively and rigorously to better understand the applicability of prediction algorithms in actual clinical practice.

So for the practicing physician, what's not to like? Where many physicians hesitate about the move to big data in clinical care, the concerns are less likely around the principle of data-driven care, but rather the manner in which these new tools are being applied. Physicians recognize the opportunity to tailor both therapeutics and improvement efforts to the product of rigorous analytics, but they likewise and uniquely understand the hazard of prematurely committing ourselves to uniform adoption of any standards. Recent findings regarding the hazards of implicit bias encoded in predictive models highlight these risks [3]. The position of physicians at the interface between science, technology and the patient compels a more visible and engaged role in applying these new capabilities.

As big data are refined for application to patient care, physicians and other clinicians must insist and engage in order to ensure that algorithms are constructed to not only apply what is known about the biology, physiology and pathology of the patient, but a more holistic view, such as is provided in an ongoing primary care relationship or even in a second opinion referral for a specialist. In these more human settings, physicians are responsible for eliciting and incorporating a much broader view of the patient and her/his life. Included in these added dimensions are considerations of values, preferences, spirituality, support, emotion, finance, anxiety and even fear, to name just a few. While elements of each could one day be incorporated in a more holistic digital view of the patient (for example, with the incorporation of survey, consumer, purchasing and social media into clinical analytics), for now these remain the domain of the human care team. Absent consideration of these elements, no artificial intelligence alone can be complete in determining a diagnosis or management plan.

Physicians and other clinical experts are also uniquely qualified to appreciate the externalities that drive clinical care and decision-making, most of which are also disarticulated from current clinical decision support tools. Issues around social determinants of health, community and social networks impact clinical decisions and resource allocation for the group of physicians particularly committed to the care of the underserved. These experts are appropriately suspect of automated tools that have not been adequately scrutinized to ensure that they have not encoded the same implicit and explicit biases that can otherwise influence policy and practice. Incomplete consideration of these important risk factors itself introduces risk to the care of these patients.

This isn't to say that it is the perspective of physicians to shelter themselves or their patients from the enormous potential benefit of big data on improved outcomes, safety, experience or value. Rather, physicians want to apply the same judicious scrutiny employed when evaluating a new therapy or treatment for our patients. Big data algorithms will not always be tested to the familiar standard of double-blinded randomized-controlled trials. However, they should be examined more critically with respect to the concerns for individual and community variation. Ideally, purveyors of these tools should be compelled to include such considerations in their products whenever possible, or at least to highlight limitations. In practice, physicians should stand guard to respond to the familiar presentations and pitches that purport to solve the biggest problems in health care and patient management with a simple app or algorithm. Skepticism on the part of physicians is as valuable now as it was in the era of the snake oil salesman.

On a more practical and immediate note, physicians need to push back against the premature and overly-strict implementation of even high quality big data tools. Specifically, organized physician groups in particular must take a firm and active stand against the universal and strict application of prediction models, clinical pathways and algorithms. While it is true that most patients can and should receive the benefit of standardized care, physicians and other clinicians need the latitude to invoke immediate and infinite variability when the circumstance warrants it, without concern for failing to achieve 100% compliance to the proscribed pathway. Personalized medicine is not consistent with 100% standardized care, so long as the variation delivered is deliberate and justified. Performance measures and incentive plans must bake this appreciation of clinical variability into their models until such time as the data and analytics truly represent the diversity of the needs and patients served.

Value

Arguably, the single biggest influence on the US health care system has been the move to value-based care. Put in its most simple and optimistic form, care delivery focused on value aspires to deliver the best possible outcome, while simultaneously balancing the expense of the care delivered. To highlight this reconciliation, value has been described in the following (over-) simplified formula:

$$\text{Value} = \frac{\text{Quality}}{\text{Expense}}$$

When expressed in this fashion, the relationship becomes clear and to some, inarguable. The delivery of high quality health care has always been of preeminent concern, not only to physicians but to all stakeholders in the care system, and especially to patients themselves! From the perspective of many physicians, however, the inclusion of expense in the equation may seem off-putting at first glance. However, as is the case for the trends and issues already discussed, the move to value will depend on a deeper engagement on the part of physicians to facilitate better understanding and alignment.

Historically, physicians, even the small business people who ran private practices, have been somewhat insulated from the challenges of our expensive health care system. Reimbursement based on the volume of care provided allowed for physicians to influence their take with a relatively simple formula: the more patients I see the more income I will generate (whether for me, my group practice or my hospital employer). Incentives were similarly aligned and so we witnessed the emergence of the physician rainmaker: the high volume specialist materially drives the bottom line for clinical business.

In an era of value-based care, this model shifts radically. In this context, physicians (and indeed the health system as a whole) are singularly aligned on the delivery of improved outcomes. Whether in the application of penalties and downside or incentives, physicians, increasingly salaried by hospitals or health systems, are compelled to provide for the highest quality of care. At the same time, those who would pay for this care (most commonly insurers, including the Federal government, but increasingly patients at risk for high-deductible coverage plans) insist that these improved outcomes be delivered for less cost.

The change can be disruptive for physicians in practice. Existing and seemingly reliable incentive and compensation models are set aside for new applications of shared services and gain sharing. Physicians are left puzzled, agitated and frequently exhausted by complex determinations of attribution, risk adjustment and performance (see section "Big Data"). With their livelihoods at stake, mistrust in the data abounds. Comprehensive reporting requirements and infrastructure needs have driven innumerable formerly independent practitioners to the arms of salaried staff positions in hospitals and health systems.

There is no denying the challenge faced by the physicians being carried if not submerged by this wave of change. However, the present state of turmoil need not be the future state. Perhaps with a dose of optimism, we can anticipate a forthcoming era in care delivery that not only allows physicians to appreciate, but even to benefit from the alignment on value. In doing so, the various trends discussed here start to come together to form a more holistic view of future practice, in which the perspective of physicians is applied more meaningfully to the benefit of patients and providers alike.

In value-based care, a premium is placed on insuring that each member of the care team is practicing at his or her highest possible scope of work. To the physician in a well-run system, historic frustration and labors around routine activities that ought to be handled by those with less training and experience (and for whom the cost of labor is much lower) are resolved once and for all. The primary care physician practices alongside medical assistants who ensure the smooth running of the operation. For the surgeon, time is spent in the operating room, practicing her unique skills absent the responsibilities assumed by the PA rounding on the follow-up patient or the clinical pharmacist ensuring medication reconciliation and education.

The electronic health record in a value environment achieves the necessary standards for interoperability and care coordination originally promised. Robust embedded registries highlight gaps in care and opportunities for improvement without relying on the dedication or memory of the physician. Doctors are left to do what they do best in interacting with patients, freed from the tyranny of the keyboard but confident that their articulated orders and expectations are captured and executed with high reliability.

Big data comes to the fore in value-based care. Progressively more robust and holistic data models incorporate greater insights into the whole patient. Routine decision-making is readily prompted for the physician, who practices with the understanding that his or her mind is freed to apply his/her knowledge with greater respect and understanding for the unique needs of the patient in front of her/him.

With a focus on wellness and outcomes, every physician's voice and significance is amplified. Profits are no longer derived solely from the volume generated by a handful of specialists and surgeons. Rather, physicians share an equitable piece of the success of the organization, reducing the sense of inequity between specialties and services. Investments are applied with a mind to promoting the health of the community served and, in doing so, can be applied with consideration also of the health and well-being of those who provide the service. Perhaps most importantly, the physicians in a value environment understand that the approach is one that addresses not only the needs of the patients before us today but also speaks for the sustainability of our entire system. The cost curve shown earlier cannot be maintained and the poor performance of our system cannot and should not be tolerated. In the successful value environment, cost savings that are accrued are not only passed on to patients (in the form of reduced health care expenditures) but are also reinvested in the system in a manner that promotes outcomes. In doing so, value-based care also expands access to care, allowing physicians and other providers to fulfill the oaths and commitments they took when they first came into practice.

A Guide for Patients

Of course, even the most detailed and optimistic aspirations for the future of American health care will not meet the immediate needs of today's patients. Pathology and physiology will not wait for the cost curve to bend, for the electronic health record to be optimized or for enhanced value to support access for all. The patients of today, whether confronting acute and life threatening illness or endeavoring to chart a course for wellness, must navigate the imperfect system and resources available to them now. So what advice can be offered to patients, families and loved ones seeking the best possible outcomes today?

The proverbial quality-seeking US health care consumer is real. You may be one yourself when choosing a physician, a health plan or a destination when in need of urgent care. When doing so, we are left to sort through incomprehensible and often conflicting ratings, rankings and performance measures in order to form an opinion of the provider we are about to encounter. How does one balance conflicting results between the Leapfrog Group and *U.S. News and World Report*? Are reviews on Yelp more significant than the number of CMS stars awarded to a provider?

Reconsideration of the themes addressed earlier in this chapter points to a framework and a more structured approach to sort through the morass of ratings and recommendations issued by the government, advertisers, third parties or even friends and neighbors. In probing for information about these factors, patients and those who would support them can apply their own values and preference to weight the information obtained. Doing so compels the health care consumer to investigation and advocacy, for such information is not always readily available or clearly presented. However, as more and more patients press for this kind of information, market forces will eventually compel both providers and provider organizations to deliver clear and authentic responses to inquiries, such as those listed below about each of these critical domains. For now though, patients and prospective patients are encouraged to pose the following and similar queries as they determine to whom they should entrust their care

- Teamwork
  - Who will be the members of my care team and what is the role of each individual?
  - How does the care team coordinate their work together in support of patients like me?
  - For how long has this team served together?
  - What activities and approaches does the team employ to ensure seamless communication and coordination of care?
- Technology
  - Which electronic health record is used in this practice and for how long has it been in place?
  - How are clinicians trained in the use of the electronic health record? Is this training refreshed periodically?
  - To what extent does the electronic health record allow for portability of my medical information? Can your EMR "talk" to other systems?
  - How do clinicians in this practice feel about the electronic health record you employ?
  - Have there been any privacy breaches involving your information management system?
  - Besides for my own care, how will my data be used?
- Data and Accountability
  - How are data employed to measure outcomes in this practice?

- Are those measures available publicly?
- Is the compensation of the physicians and other team members tied to measureable outcomes? Are they incentivized for healthy patients or for the amount of testing or treatment that you provide?
- Did physicians and other clinicians take part in selecting the metrics on which their compensation is based?
- Value
  - How does this practice/institution ensure that physicians and other members of the care team are appropriately using resources in the management of patients?
  - Are physicians incentivized to reduce or control costs without regard to clinical outcomes?
  - Do the members of the clinical team here each practice to the highest scope of his/her license and ability?
  - Are physicians and other clinicians participants in managing the budget and expenditures of this practice/institution?

Conclusions

This chapter began with a pessimistic perspective on the state of health care in the United States. For all of the achievements in clinical care, biomedical discovery and education of the next generation of clinicians, our current delivery system does not yet deliver as we wish it would. That being said, our course forward to meet even the most ambitious of aspirations seems in some respects very clear. Physicians, through training, experience, values and character, must have the opportunity to uniquely and fundamentally determine the future effectiveness of American health care. Authentic partnerships with other stakeholders, in which the voice of physicians is heard but never supersedes the needs of patients, will be critical. Teamwork, judicious application of technology, robust analytics, patient engagement and a deep commitment to providing value in order to support access together serve as the foundation of this effort. In this manner, the perspective of the physician is not just instructive, but the essential first step to delivering the care delivery system to which we all aspire and that our patients deserve.

References

1. Ofri D. The business of health care depends on exploiting doctors and nurses. The New York Times. Sept 6, 2019. Accessed online Feb 14, 2020.
2. Tawfik DS, Profit J, Morgenthaler TI, Satele DV, Sinsky CA, Dyrbye LN, Tutty MA, West CP, Shanafelt TD. Physician burnout, well-being, and work unit safety grades in relationship to reported medical errors. Mayo Clin Proc. 2018;93(11):1571–80.
3. Rajkomar A, Hardt M, Howell MD, Corrado G, Chin MH. Ensuring fairness in machine learning to advance health equity. Ann Intern Med. 2018;169(12):866–72.

Voice of the Nurse

3

Debra Albert and Sally Walton

Nursing Practice

Nurses are the largest component of the health care delivery system and are present in most all care settings. Despite this fact, often the practice of nursing is not well understood, and thus this role is not fully used as a source of reference and point of contact for patients as they traverse the health care system. To understand the potential and how this role can further benefit patients, clear understanding of the professional practice is important. The *Nursing Scope and Standards of Practice* and the *Code of Ethics for Nurses with Interpretive Statements* collectively guide nursing practice in all roles and settings [1].

Nursing Scope and Standards of Practice

The American Nurses Association (ANA) [1] model of professional nursing practice regulation originated from the ANA and guides nursing practice discussions. The model illustrates four levels of standards, regulations, policies, and autonomy nurses should adhere to within their practice. Nurses must incorporate all of these levels into their practice, along with the use of evidence, to achieve the goal of safe and quality nursing practice. Additionally, health care nursing leadership must align their goals and mission with quality and safety to support consistent practice in all areas and at all levels [2].

Within the *Nursing Scope and Standards of Practice*, standard 14 "Quality of Practice" focuses on how the nurses contribute to quality of nursing practice. This

D. Albert (✉) · S. Walton
University of Chicago, Chicago, IL, USA
e-mail: Debra.Albert@nyulangone.org; Sally.Walton@uchospitals.edu

© Springer Nature Switzerland AG 2020
P. V. Sreeramoju et al. (eds.), *The Patient and Health Care System: Perspectives on High-Quality Care*, https://doi.org/10.1007/978-3-030-46567-4_3

standard states that the skills of the nurse include the ability to recognize challenges and opportunities, along with proposing ways to improve nursing quality. The nurse participates both independently, and with a multidisciplinary team, in the collection and analysis of data to track nursing quality [1].

Nurses also create, contribute to, and revise policies and processes for improving care quality to ensure that the care is supported by proper documentation. In the role as a leader, nurses contribute to quality improvement, project development, and translating the evidence or research results and known best practices into practice by applying knowledge at the point of care, which improves patient outcomes [1].

Code of Ethics for Nurses with Interpretive Statements

Many provisions within the *Code of Ethics for Nurses with Interpretive Statements* reference the nurses' obligations to ensure quality care. These include provisions that describe application of nursing standards and guidelines, assessment of quality improvement initiatives, monitoring activities, and evaluating outcomes and quality of care they provide or delegated to other health care providers [3].

According to the ANA [3], to achieve this, nurses must work autonomously, as well as collaboratively, to maintain an environment conducive to ongoing quality and to meet common goals of delivering efficient and effective quality care. Environments that foster ongoing quality are those in which professional voices of nurses are valued and responded to. These environments foster teamwork and inter-disciplinary communication that happens openly, timely, and remains focused on patient needs. Nurses must also plan to provide high-quality, patient-specific health care in collaboration with, and through the influence and guidance of, other health care professionals [3]. This planning most often includes interdisciplinary care planning, in which the short-term and long-term needs of the patient is discussed with each clinician contributing knowledge and information which the entire team uses to ensure the most individualized and effective plan. Many health care organizations have created ways to include the patient and the patient's family in this care planning process. Ensuring patient involvement in this process is a best practice to ensure care decision actively involves the patient's wishes and values.

According to Sherwood [2], "Quality improvement uses data to monitor outcomes of care processes that help guide improvement methods to design and test changes in the system to continuously improve outcomes". Through ongoing quality monitoring and collaboration between health care professionals and patients, health care organizations are transformed. This process exemplifies working toward a common goal that leads to better health, better care, and better professional advancement [2].

Nurse executives are responsible for facilitating nursing's inclusion in organizational quality and safety councils to ensure active engagement in discussion and decisions that may affect care they provide to patients; thus, recognizing the nurses value as a clinical expert [3].

Moving Nursing Care Forward

Current State of Health Care Quality

Fifteen years after the National Academy of Medicine's (NAM) publication of *To Err is Human: Building a Safer Health System*, the urgency for improvement that was originally created, has now slowed, yet the state of quality and safety in health care continues to demand our attention [4]. We continue to hear about medical errors in the media, along with the perception of the absence of organizational accountability to provide quality care, and the public is becoming more dissatisfied [4]. Exploration into quality of care reveals that change is slow, new problems develop, costs are higher, regulatory requirements are more rigorous, and performance on many quality indicators has remained stagnant or gotten worse over the last 10 years [4]. For these reasons, engaging patients in their care and decision-making process also requires our ongoing attention.

According to Sherwood [2], if health care professionals feel that they are unable to provide good care, morale and job satisfaction may be affected. Quality is an essential value and nursing professionals take pride in doing the right thing for patients; nevertheless, quality care is more than wanting to do the right thing. Quality care involves the ability to use information and tools to guide analysis of processes to improve systems [2]. As care providers, it is essential for nurses and other clinicians to remember that patients are the final evaluators of quality care. As such, elements of service, such as patient experience, are included in improvement efforts.

It is vital for nurses to be accountable for translating evidence into health care practice and the NAM recommends four key strategies to improve the quality of care and safety for patient. These include establishing a national focus to create leadership research tools and practices to increase the understanding of safety, develop a national, public incident reporting system and encourage organizations to participate and voluntarily report, improve standards and expectations for safety improvements and apply safety systems to ensure safe practice at the bedside [4].

Gaps in Health Care Quality

The NAM's other report, *Crossing the Quality Chasm: A New Health System for the 21st Century*, identifies that health care delivery is deficient in its ability to actually translate knowledge into practice and safely apply new technologies. Further, the NAM describes six goals for the improvement of health care, which are to ensure it is safe, timely, effective, efficient, equitable, and patient-centered [4]. Nurses can and do play a role in each of these goals. For example, safe care is care that protects patients from medical errors and does not cause harm; this can be demonstrated through the nurses' role in medication administration. The nurse can practice safe care by ensuring application of the "five rights" of medication administration and ensuring proper use of medication safety technology, such as automated medication dispensing cabinets and barcode medication administration (BCMA). Also, patient-centered care is care that is responsive to a patient's needs and preferences. Examples include the nurse ensuring physical comfort for patients through effective pain management and/or assistance with activities of daily living (ADL's), as well as meeting a patient's request to be fully informed about their clinical status and plan of care.

According to Sherwood [2], most industries that have seen vast improvements in quality have one overarching agency that sets the expectations. However in health care, that responsibility is spread among various agencies and none of them include a purpose of gathering quality data for broad analysis and dissemination [2]. Unfortunately, a centralized, national infrastructure to implement these strategies does not exist; yet quality and safety experts continue to work on strategies to address the NAM recommendations [4].

Quality and Safety Experts' Strategies for Improving Health Care Quality

The Joint Commission established the National Patient Safety Goals in 2002, which are evidence-based quality and safety strategies that integrate the best available scientific evidence with the best available experiential evidence [5]. They provide recommendations for high vulnerability areas (i.e. medication safety, patient identification, infection prevention), as well as offer proven solutions by examining systematic processes for quality improvement, patient safety and measuring outcomes [5]. Following these recommendations, nurses and the organizations they work in focus on creating routine methods to increase patient safety. These efforts include medication labeling and administration techniques requiring two nurses to verify for certain high risk medications, ensuring accurate patient identification, routine hand washing, and engaging patients and families in efforts to reduce patient falls as some examples.

The Patient Safety and Quality Improvement Act of 2005 is a national law with a goal to make it easier for providers to report and learn from medical errors through becoming Patient Safety Organizations (PSOs) [6]. According to the Agency for Health Care Research and Quality (AHRQ) [6], there are 88 PSOs that are certified by the AHRQ, as of December 2019. The AHRQ is working to develop systematic methods to learn from the data collected by PSOs to improve care [6].

According to White et al. [4], public reporting of hospital quality data is increasing. Quality leaders in the industry, such as the Institute for Health Care Improvement (IHI), continue to highlight quality and safety issues. The IHI developed the Triple Aim framework which focuses on providing better quality care and better patient experience, improving the health of people and communities and affordable care [7].

Business groups such as Leapfrog align their standards for hospital performance and strive to push for quality and safety transparency in the U.S. health system [8]. Safety ratings from Leapfrog are given to acute-care hospitals in the United States twice a year and this rating is starting to be considered a "gold standard" for hospital patient safety [8]. These standards focus on governance and leadership accountability, structural and process components that enable a culture of safety and organizational resource allocation to support this important work.

As the largest and most commonly present component of the health care system, nurses are closest to this essential work regardless of setting, regardless of patient population, and regardless of delivery model. As such, nurses must be involved in these efforts to lead transformation.

Improving Health Care Quality through Implementation of Evidence

One way to approach implementation of evidence is through frameworks or models of translation. One example is The Comprehensive Unit-based Safety Program (CUSP), which is a patient safety model created through a collaborative effort of the AHRQ and national patient safety leaders; it is a model that deems harm is not "an acceptable cost of doing business" [9]. It consists of five basic steps: educate in safety science, identify defects, engage executive leaders, learn from defects, and implementing work tools [9].

According to the Agency for Health Care Research and Quality [9], it is a technique that can help clinical teams provide safer care by uniting best practices and the science of safety. The CUSP "Stories of Success: Using CUSP To Improve Safety" report shows how hospitals have applied CUSP to improve care [10].

Professional Nursing Organizations Working Toward Improving Health Care Quality

Professional nursing organizations have also made recommendations to improve quality of care. For example, the American Nurses Credentialing Center (ANCC) Magnet Recognition program standards are based on quality improvement and recognize quality in nursing care delivery [2].

The ANA established the National Database of Nursing Quality Indicators (NDNQI), which maintains comparative data on performance in nursing sensitive indicators, such as falls, staffing, and restraints [11]. This large national database is a key resource, as nurses at all levels of the health care system work to improve patient care. By providing meaningful comparisons on key outcomes of nursing care, this data base often serves as a source of information as nurses seek to understand the impact of their care and opportunities to improve that. While all levels of the nursing team access and use this data, it is most powerful when bedside clinical nurses understand and apply the data directly.

The Nursing Alliance for Quality Care was formed to bring a unified nursing perspective to ensure: (1) patients receive the right care, at the right time, by the right licensed personnel, (2) nurses advocate for and are accountable to high quality care that is patient-centered, and (3) the recognition of the role of nurses in high quality, patient-centered care by policymakers [2].

NAM recommends three central principles nurses can use to lead change. First, nurses must have insight to recognize quality and safety care and issues in their daily work. Second, transforming education programs to address quality competencies to help with knowledge, skills, and attitudes. Third, determining best practices and how to establish and apply evidence-based, systematic approaches to transform health care [2].

Nursing Education to Improve Quality

Nursing professionals must have the proper education and training to facilitate this ability to improve care and systems to an extent that quality improvement becomes part of their daily work. Nursing professional education has undergone some modifications to improve care by better preparing nurses in quality and safety education using knowledge, skills, and attitudes [2]. These modifications have happened over a number of years and in multiple phases first focused on nursing education at the point of entering the profession and now through graduate and postgraduate education [12].

Quality and Safety Education for Nurses

The Quality and Safety Education for Nurses (QSEN) [13] project "addresses the challenge of preparing future nurses with the knowledge, skills, and attitudes (KSAs) necessary to continuously improve the quality and safety of the health care systems within which they work". The aim of QSEN is to "educate the nursing workforce to be competent in patient safety and health care quality principles" [14]. A goal for QSEN is to change nurses' approach to practice based on inquiry and how to make care better, design and use evidence-based standards, examine outcomes and errors from a system perspective, and work in multidisciplinary care delivery teams [2]. The QSEN competences include: patient-centered care, teamwork and collaboration, evidence-based practice, quality improvement, safety, and informatics [15].

According to Cronenwett et al. [16], nurses need to be prepared with a set of competencies using evidence allowing them to describe what makes up good care, identify gaps in care, and to know what they could do to close those gaps; these competencies define what it means to be a respected and qualified nurse. At the core of nursing is the passion and will to ensure quality and safety for patients and this value in quality is evident in numerous nursing publications, the standards of practice, and accreditation guidelines discussed.

Quality Improvement

The quality improvement competencies help prepare nurses to participate in quality improvement as part of their daily work. These competencies also address the gaps for executing on a nursing quality and safety curriculum. Knowledge includes strategies for learning about care outcomes of clinical practice, including under-standing the critical role nurses play as part of the care system, and how nursing processes affect patient outcomes. This knowledge is also key to understanding the importance of consistent measurement in evaluating quality of care and making recommendations for altering care processes [16].

The skills include using information about patient populations and aligning qual-ity improvement initiatives to address them [16]. Skills also include the use of tools to guide care processes, participate in Root Cause Analysis (RCA) activities, the use of measures to understand performance and identify gaps in practice in order to align goals and metrics to improve care and finally be able to evaluate the extent of change [16].

The attitudes are described by Cronenwett et al. [16] as nurses recognizing that though their essential daily work includes continuous quality improvement, they must also value everyone's contribution to patient care outcomes. Additionally, nurses must realize how inconsistency in practice affects care, but also realize the "joy" in the work they do and appreciate what all team members bring to improve care [16].

Safety

The goal of the safety competency is to "minimize risk of harm to patients and pro-viders through both system effectiveness and individual performance" [15]. Within the safety competency is knowledge related to examining elements that create a culture of safety and Just Culture, finding an operational approach to support a high reliability organization and illustrate best practices in response to errors/near misses/good catches.

The skills related to safety are the use of evidence-based practice to further Just Culture, the reporting of errors/good catches, encouraging nurses to report and the development of policies to guide response to errors/near misses/good catches. The attitudes related to safety are the use of a systems approach to enhancing patient care, promoting error reporting as the foundational component to improve quality and the use of error reporting systems [15].

Barriers to Implementing Evidence-Based Care

Throughout this chapter, the concept of applying research outcomes or evidence and best practices has been stressed as a key to improving the quality of patient care and outcomes. However, this is far more complex than might be appreciated. The first barrier to consider is the nursing profession itself. There are several million nurses working in America with different education levels, specializations, work settings, skill and experience levels, familiarity with research, time spent studying, as well as racial and ethnic backgrounds. This heterogeneity most certainly impacts imple-mentation of new knowledge into practice [17].

The context of the suggested practice change also impacts how easily and quickly the change is implanted into routine care process. Specifically, the extent to which the nurse understands and has confidence in the change are key determining factors. One key factor in facilitating change is understanding how it fits with current practice. Additional factors include the nursing culture, the size of the organization, support for nurses to access research findings, access to content experts, time to devote to such work, and provision of education on change and implementation processes [17].

Overcoming these barriers takes commitment and resources both from the nursing profession and the organizations in which they work. As the largest group of direct care providers, nurses are positioned to be key drivers in evidence implementation. However, to lead this work, nursing education must include evidence implementation in formal undergraduate and graduate programs of study. Education at both levels will ensure that new nurses have the skills they need to effectively participate in improving care and that nurse leaders and clinical experts at the graduate level can lead such work within the interdisciplinary team. Health care organizations must consider increasing advanced nursing roles focused on implementation and improvement science. These roles are aimed at bringing the research findings and practice improvements to the daily care routines of nurses. Such roles serve as content experts and resources for bedside clinical staff in improvement efforts [18]. An example of how important such investments are in improving patient care outcomes is the role of Skin Care experts. While this role may be titled differently, most organizations have such a role. The nurses in this role are responsible for remaining up-to-date on any changes in the standard of care in pressure ulcer prevention methods. These nurses often lead groups of bedside nurses and help to develop this specialized skill set in an identified group of nurses. These nurses, in turn, serve as unit or department internal experts for their peers working in the same unit or department. Thus, with a small investment of one skin care nurse expert, this expertise and application of specialized knowledge is multiplied several times over and thus, therefore, improving the care to all patients served in the organization.

Where Do We Go from Here?

Clearly, there is much work to be done, as health care in general and the nursing profession work to create safer and more effective care accessible for all patients. And, while this is a never-ending pursuit of quality improvement, there are some concrete steps that key stakeholder groups can take now to support this work. One publication that provides critical and foundational guidance is the 2010 National Academy of Medicine report, The Future of Nursing: Leading Change [19]. This report identified eight nationally focused recommendations and defined specific actions for key groups to achieve these. As of this writing, many of these recommendations are not or will not be achieved. Some specific examples of these are: Expand opportunities for nurses to lead and diffuse collaborative improvement efforts, Increase the proportion of nurses with a baccalaureate degree to 80% by 2020, and Prepare and enable nurses to lead change to advance health. As a subset of the full list of recommendations, looking at these three examples, it is easy to see the need for broad-based action by various groups to effect such change.

Expanding opportunities for nurses to lead and diffuse collaborative improvement efforts includes efforts to conduct research and redesign or improve practice environments. To this end, government agencies should ensure nurses are included in leadership roles in efforts to evaluate models of payment and care delivery. Performance measures that reflect the impact of nursing in quality patient care should be identified and implemented. Funding sources, public and private, should support nursing research to enable nursing contributions to improved health care outcomes. And health care organizations, as the most common employer of nurses, should include clinical nurses, from all care settings, in all product purchase and implementation and evaluation of relevant product and technology decisions. They should also support nurses in developing, adopting, and evaluating new models of patient care [19]. In 2010, 76 articles published in the top 10 health services research journals were coauthored by a registered nurse. While that number increased to an all-time high of 134 articles in 2014, there has since been a trend downward to only 71 coauthored research journal published articles in 2017 [20].

Increasing the proportion of nurses with a baccalaureate degree to 80% by 2020 will require collaboration and partnership of nursing education accrediting bodies and providers, funding sources, and employers to increase access to higher levels of nursing education and to support a more diversified nursing workforce. Specifically, further collaboration among nursing schools, as directed by accrediting bodies, would provide access to higher levels of education through academic pathways supporting educational advancement. Employers should offer tuition reimbursement to clinical nurses, helping to move diploma and associate degree nurses to baccalaureate levels. Additionally, supporting and offering continuing education support enables nurses to maintain educational advancements. Governmental agencies, such as the Health Resources and Services Administration, as well as private and public funders, should expand or create grant or loan programs to encourage higher education and targeted to populations to diversify the nursing workforce. And finally, nursing schools should partner with other health profession schools to build joint educational offerings into curriculum aimed at teaching and reinforcing interprofessional education [19]. While the goal of this recommendation is 80% by 2020, the starting level was 49% in 2010. As of July 2019, the most updated national baccalaureate rate was 56% [21] and this recommendation will not be achieved by 2020.

Preparing and enabling nurses to lead change and advance health focuses on how nurses are prepared for this work and what opportunities exist for nurses. Nurses must take responsibility for professional growth and seek out opportunities to develop leadership skills offering to lead performance improvement initiatives. Nursing education must include leadership content in formal curriculum, while nurse leaders and nursing associations must role model and provide mentorship opportunities for clinical nurses as they develop these skills. Health care decision makers, governmental, public, and private, must include nursing representation on boards and other key leadership decision-making bodies [19]. The goal for this recommendation is to have 10,000 nurses serving on various boards. As of July 2019, only 6311 nurses report this activity [21]. More alarming is the look at boards of hospitals, which are the largest employers of nurses. In 2011, 6% of hospital boards had a registered nurse member. In 2018, only 4% reported this representation! [20]

It is essential that nurses understand, provide leadership by example and promote the importance of providing quality health care [14].

References

1. American Nurses Association. Nursing scope and standards of practice. 3rd ed. Silver Spring: ANA; 2015b.
2. Sherwood G. Driving forces for quality and safety: changing mindsets to improve health care. In: Sherwood G, Barnsteiner J, editors. Quality and safety in nursing: a competency approach to improving outcomes. Hoboken: Wiley Blackwell; 2017. p. 3–20. Retrieved from https://www.psnet.ahrq.gov/issue/quality-and-safety-nursing-competency-approach-improving-outcomes-second-edition.
3. American Nurses Association. Code of ethics for nurses with interpretive statements. 2015a. Retrieved from https://www.nursingworld.org/coe-view-only.
4. White KM, Dudley-Brown S, Terhaar MF. Translation of evidence into nursing and health care. New York: Springer Publishing; 2016.
5. The Joint Commission. 2019 Hospital National Patient Safety Goals. 2019. Retrieved from https://www.jointcommission.org/assets/1/6/2019_HAP_NPSGs_final2.pdf.
6. Agency for Healthcare Research and Quality. Patient Safety Organization (PSO) program. 2019. Retrieved December 26, 2019 from https://pso.ahrq.gov/listed.
7. Institute for Healthcare Improvement. The IHI triple aim. 2019. Retrieved from http://www.ihi.org/Engage/Initiatives/TripleAim/Pages/default.aspx.
8. Leapfrog Hospitals Safety Grade. About the grade. 2019. Retrieved from https://www.hospitalsafetygrade.org/your-hospitals-safety-grade/about-the-grade.
9. Agency for Healthcare Research and Quality. The CUSP method. 2018. Retrieved from https://www.ahrq.gov/professionals/education/curriculum-tools/cusptoolkit/index.html.
10. Agency for Healthcare Research and Quality. Stories of success: using CUSP to improve safety. 2012. Retrieved from https://www.ahrq.gov/sites/default/files/publications/files/cusp-success.pdf.
11. National Database of Nursing Quality Indicators. NDNQI nursing-sensitive indicators. 2019. Retrieved from https://nursingandndnqi.weebly.com/ndnqi-indicators.html.
12. Kelly P, Vottero B, Christie-McAuliffe C. Introduction to quality and safety education for nurses. New York: Springer Publishing; 2014.
13. Quality and Safety Education for Nurses. About QSEN. 2018. Retrieved from http://qsen.org/about-qsen/.
14. Lyle-Edrosolo G, Waxman KT. Aligning Healthcare Safety and Quality competencies: Quality and Safety Education for Nurses (QSEN), The Joint Commission, and The American Nurses Credentialing Center (ANCC) Magnet Standards Crosswalk. 2016. Retrieved from https://doi.org/10.1016/j.mnl.2015.08.005.
15. American Association of Colleges of Nursing. QSEN education consortium. Graduate-level QSEN competencies: knowledge, skills and attitudes. 2012. Retrieved from http://www.aacnnursing.org/Portals/42/AcademicNursing/CurriculumGuidelines/Graduate-QSEN-Competencies.pdf.

16. Cronenwett LR, Sherwood GD, Barnsteiner JH, Disch J, Johnson J, Mitchell PH, Sullivan D, Warren JJ. Quality and safety education for nurses. Nurs Outlook. 2007;55(3):122–31. https://doi.org/10.1016/j.outlook.2007.02.006.
17. van Achterberg T, Schoonhoven L, Grol R. Nursing implementation science: how evidence-based nursing requires evidenced-based implementation. J Nurs Scholarsh. 2008;40(4):302–10.
18. Flynn R, Scott S, Rotter T, Hartfield D. The potential for nurses to contribute to and lead improvement science in health care. J Adv Nurs. 2016;73(1):97–107.
19. Institute of Medicine (US) Committee on the Robert Wood Johnson Foundation Initiative on the Future of Nursing, at the Institute of Medicine. The future of nursing: leading change. Advancing health report recommendations. 2011. Retrieved July 1, 2017, from https://pubmed.ncbi.nlm.nih.gov/24983041/.
20. Campaign for Action. Dashboard secondary indicator. 2019b. Retrieved July 18, 2019, from https://campaignforaction.org.
21. Campaign for Action. Welcome to the future of nursing. Campaign for Action dashboard. 2019a. Retrieved July 18, 2019, from https://campaignforaction.org.

Part II

Current Landscape

The Quality Landscape

William G. Reed

Quality of health care and patient safety have become important topics in the public and medical press of the United States since the publication of *To Err is Human* almost two decades ago. This is not surprising since that publication reported two studies confirming that medical errors and preventable harm from medical treatment contribute substantially to morbidity and mortality in the United States accounting for an estimated 44,000–98,000 deaths per year [1]. Unfortunately, little progress has been made over the past two decades in reversing this trend despite efforts to increase the understanding of why it is occurring. The delivery of health care is very complicated and sick patients have a high risk for complications and death, no matter what is done. However, medicine's efforts to reduce these numbers have stalled, while other professions that deal with dangerous situations, such as aviation, have improved safety tremendously over the past few decades. The purpose of this chapter is to provide a perspective on the current status of health care quality in the United States.

What Is Quality in Health Care?

Quality in health care was defined by the National Academy of Medicine as "the degree to which health services for individuals and populations increase the likelihood of desired health outcomes and are consistent with current professional knowledge" [1] (Fig. 4.1). This definition emphasizes the obligation the health care system has to individual and populations of patients to improve health outcomes by

W. G. Reed (✉)
Department of Internal Medicine, UT Southwestern Medical Center,
Dallas, TX, USA

Quality, Safety and Outcomes Education, UT Southwestern Medical Center,
Dallas, TX, USA
e-mail: Gary.Reed@UTSouthwestern.edu

© Springer Nature Switzerland AG 2020
P. V. Sreeramoju et al. (eds.), *The Patient and Health Care System: Perspectives on High-Quality Care*, https://doi.org/10.1007/978-3-030-46567-4_4

Fig. 4.1 Quality in health care

The degree to which health services for individuals and populations increase the likelihood of desired health outcomes and are consistent with current professional knowledge.

Fig. 4.2 Health care quality

Safe

Timely

Effective

Efficient

Equitable

Patient-centered

providing care consistent with published best practices. Outcomes of care are the primary determinants of quality against which all care must be measured. This emphasis on process of care outcomes is important, as new treatment and care options are developed.

The National Academy of Medicine also defined several components of quality that should be considered when measuring the quality of health care [2] (Fig. 4.2). These components of quality include the entire spectrum of health care delivery. Understanding the relationships among these components is critical to improving overall health care quality because it means the traditional "silos" of responsibility and accountability in health care have to be dismantled for quality and safety to be maximally improved. While these silos are understandable, given the reductionism emphasized by medical research over the last century, they inhibit the ability to look at quality at a system or macro level. For example, a health care system may provide low-cost care to a group of patients, but the care is substandard according to published best practices. Should this system be rewarded in our payment system? Most would think not.

The delivery of medical care should be thought of as a system and judged by the total outcomes of that system, not individual domains within the system.

However, the six domains of quality illustrated above provide a useful framework to judge the total quality of a health care system when taken as a whole. First, the care must be safe. This domain is probably the most important. A tenet of medicine is to "first, do no harm" and providing safe care is a moral obligation of our system. Second, the care should be timely. This means that the care should be given when the patient needs it and not at the convenience of the care delivery system. Many times, this domain is measured in terms of access to care by patients or populations of patients. Next, the care should be effective. This means that the care delivered should be consistent with best medical practices. Unfortunately, much of the care delivered in the US health system is based on tradition and not based on evidence from medical research. The domain of efficiency brings in the variable of cost to the quality equation. Health care should be delivered at the lowest necessary cost,

Fig. 4.3 Value in   Value = (Quality + Access + Experience)/ Expense
health care

not the lowest possible cost to avoid affecting the safety of the care delivered. The next domain is equity. This means that the care delivered to all patients should be based on need and not based on arbitrary variables such as insurance status, race, or other patient characteristics. This domain has been one with which the US health system has struggled and has led to many described medical disparities among those in our county. Finally, the care should be patient-centered. This means that the focus of patient care should always be on the needs of the patient and not on the needs of providers or the system of delivery of the care.

Today, the "value" of health care is considered one of the most important characteristics of the US health care system to be evaluated by the public and policymakers. Value is defined as the quality or outcomes of care (some would add access and experience here while some would argue they are included in quality) divided by the cost of the care provided (Fig. 4.3). Evaluating the "value" emphasizes the important relationship between efficiency and cost to quality and the critical perspective of patients and payers in any discussion of the quality of health care.

Another complementary model of health care value, known as the Triple Aim, has been suggested by Berwick et al. [3]. This model emphasizes the importance of improving the patient experience or quality of care, improving the health of populations and reducing the per capita cost of care as the ultimate goals of health care delivery.

Health care delivery in the United States is among the best and worst in the world, depending on the characteristic(s) examined. For example, the number of patients who suffer preventable harm each year in the United States is much too high, and the cost of health care in the United States is the highest in the world in both absolute dollars spent per capita and percent of the gross domestic product [4]. In 2016, spending per capita in the United States was just over $10,000, which is the most of any other country by far.

This high cost of health care in the United States, combined with poor outcomes in certain areas, such as preventive care, lead some to believe the value of health care in the United States is far below other developed countries [5] such as France, Canada, and the United Kingdom. On the other hand, the United States is at or near the top of the world in outcomes of certain conditions, such as cancer or major trauma. Also, we are a world leader in new technology and drug development. Patients in the United States also wait less time for elective surgery or needed consultation from a specialist than in France, Canada, the United Kingdom, and many other industrialized countries [6, 7].

In summary, the measurement of the quality of health care is very complicated, and many factors should be included. Although the National Academy of Medicine has tried to create an accepted definition of quality, others continue to use their definitions, which are frequently biased, for marketing or other propriety reasons. Focusing on a single or few factors will not give an accurate picture of quality to patients or the public.

Fig. 4.4 Safety in   Freedom from accidental injury when interacting in any way with
health care   the health care system

Safety in US Health Care

Quality of health care has an important component of patient safety at its core. The National Academy of Medicine defines safety in health care as "freedom from accidental injury when interacting in any way with the health care system" [1] (Fig. 4.4). Providing a safe environment for our patients, including the safe delivery of care, is a moral obligation of our health care system.

Over the past two decades, the discussion of patient safety in health care in the United States has become important for several inter-related reasons. First, the complexity of care delivery is much greater than in the past, increasing the risk for complications and errors. Early studies of medical errors estimated that 44,000–98,000 patients die every year in the United States from these medically related errors [8, 9], and recent studies indicate this number may be even higher. Many of these errors are due to subtle variations in practice or subconscious slips in the delivery of care and are not due to negligence or malpractice. Second, highly publicized errors have informed the public of the risks of medical errors. These errors are frequently highly sensationalized by the press, which leads to an appropriate heightened awareness of the risks of medical errors, but encourages blaming individuals for the errors rather than the system or environment in which they work. Third, payment for medical care in the United States has previously been determined primarily by the quantity or utilization of medical care, not its quality or appropriateness. In the future, programs such as Value-Based Purchasing by the Medicare System will change this, as payers convert to payment systems that reward high quality and appropriate care. It is hoped that these payment systems will more appropriately emphasize high-quality, safe, and appropriate care. Finally and most importantly, improving the quality and safety of health care is a moral obligation of health care providers to their patients.

Why Has the Health Care Industry Been Reluctant to Aggressively and Transparently Address the Issues of Quality and Safety in Health Care?

The answer to this question is complex. The mission of medicine is to help people, and those who work in health care strive to improve the lives of patients and relieve their suffering. This mission is noble and is what motivates the vast majority of people who enter the health care profession. However, the practice of medicine is inherently risky for patients, and those in the medical field deal with probabilities, not certainty, most of the time. The human body's response to many outside influences, such as disease or the treatments for disease, is not 100% predictable, and this unpredictability must be considered when evaluating the quality of care. This uncertainty is compounded by the fact that outcomes of patient care may vary based on small differences in care delivery at many levels. This *variation in care* is much of what is wrong with medical care in its current state and accounts for much of the differences in quality seen today from one practitioner or health system to another. Reducing variation in practice and care-delivery processes is an important goal for improving the quality of health care in the United States, and a complete understanding of the methodology of process improvement is critical if substantial improvements are to be made in the effectiveness of medical care.

However, medicine and the societal culture of the United States have created an environment that is not conducive to aggressively addressing the issues of quality and patient safety that exist today (Fig. 4.5). This environment is complex and has several negative drivers such as the traditional payment system that fosters overutilization and focuses on the quantity of care delivered rather than quality. In the traditional payment system in the United States, hospitals and providers were paid more if more care was delivered regardless of the need, appropriateness, or cause for the extra care. For example, a hospital would be paid a certain amount (x dollars) for the admission of a healthy patient to have their gallbladder removed. If, during that hospitalization, the patient had a urinary catheter placed, and due to improper care of the catheter, suffered a catheter-associated urinary tract infection, the hospital would be paid more ($x + y$ dollars) even though the hospital-acquired infection was preventable. This payment structure, and the belief that such complications were a normal risk of care, created a disincentive for hospitals to aggressively prevent such complications.

Also, the provision of medical care is dependent on a highly skilled workforce that, while critical to the delivery of high-quality care, fosters the erroneous belief that skilled workers are immune to human error. Skill and education do not protect one from human error, although the types of error may be different for a skilled worker when compared to an unskilled one. This misconception has led many in medicine to resist the use of simple tools, such as checklists, that have been shown to reduce errors in skilled as well as unskilled professionals.

Another challenge to the aggressive approach to quality is the belief that any improvement in quality requires a net investment of money resulting in more expensive health care. While quality improvement does frequently involve an initial investment, savings from improved care due to fewer complications, less reworking,

Fig. 4.5 Why the reluctance to address issues of quality and safety today?

Reimbursement structure of health care

Dependence on highly skilled work force

Belief that quality improvement always cost money

"Culture of blame"

Tendency to look at errors as individual failure instead of system failures

Belief that some complications are "normal"

Medical legal environment

Media obsession with sensationalism and language used

and increased efficiency more than make up the initial investment required to start the process.

A "Culture of Blame" in which the blaming of providers for mistakes is perceived to lessen the likelihood of those mistakes recurring in the future exists in many health systems across the country. This faulty logic ignores the evidence that system factors contribute, at least in part, to almost all medical errors, and these factors are frequently completely out of the control of the person blamed for the error. Unfortunately, this culture often results in hiding mistakes to avoid being caught and appearing incompetent. On a positive note, many health care systems are adopting a more evidence-based, algorithmic approach to personal culpability when a human medical error is committed. An example of more enlightened approaches to human error can be found in the writings of James Reason and the program known as "Just Culture." Hopefully, adoption of these and similar approaches will allow a more open discussion of medical error.

Traditional medical teaching has also contributed, in some part, to the reluctance to address quality issues. In the past, this style of teaching was frequently adversarial, and the demand for excellence was interpreted as a demand for perfection. Consequently, providers frequently associated human error with incompetence. Although this notion is antithetical to modern theories and evidence of human error, many are reluctant to admit even trivial errors for fear of being accused of incompetence or needing additional training to maintain competence. Fortunately, many now accept the notion that humans make errors, and we need patient safety systems that acknowledge this fact. Developing systems that mitigate and recognize human error in time to prevent the error from reaching a patient is much more effective than demanding human perfection which is unrealistic. Certainly this does not mean that diligence and striving for perfection should not be the aspirations of all providers. It does mean that we should recognize that human errors will eventually occur despite our diligence. Finally, society, in general, has contributed substantially to the current medical culture through medico-legal actions.

While this list is not complete, it does provide some of the reasons that the medical system has avoided an aggressive approach to improving quality of care and human error until recently.

Transparency and the Quality of Health Care in the United States

The past two decades have seen a shift in the health care industry toward more transparency of measures of quality of care for health systems, hospitals, clinics, and individual practitioners. This shift began with the Centers for Medicare and Medicaid Service (CMS) when it started public reporting of quality and safety metrics for US hospitals in its Hospital Compare website in 2005. The first metrics published for the public were a group of process measures called "Core Measures" and a few outcome measures such as mortality rates for patients admitted to the hospital with heart attack, congestive heart failure, and pneumonia. Since that time, other measures have been added by CMS, including some for clinics and individual practitioners, and other outcome measures, such as readmission rates and outcome of some surgical procedures. In addition, patient satisfaction scores for hospitals (HCAHPS) were added in 2008.

The public announcement of the quality measures was met with both praise and criticism from the health care industry. Most believe that patients have a right to know the level of quality delivered by individual providers so that they can make rational choices about care for themselves and their families. Reliance on individual health care systems or individual hospitals to report their quality measures was felt to be inadequate and filled with too many biases to be reliable.

However, others appropriately argue that publically reported measures are not always an accurate way to compare one system to another because some hospitals and practitioners treat sicker patients than others, and these differences in patient populations are not always reflected in the publically available quality metrics. Also, many public quality assessments of health systems have been performed by proprietary organizations, such as U.S News and World Reports™, Leapfrog™, Healthgrades™, Becker's Health Care™, Consumer Reports™, etc. While these provide insight for patients in choosing a system for care, their lack of transparency in risk-adjustment and evaluation criteria often result in marked variation in the measurement of health care systems when one method is compared to another. In fact, studies have shown that different quality assessment groups rarely agree on which hospitals deliver the best care. In addition, many of these groups use their quality ratings to sell consulting services to organizations that want to improve their ratings. Others allow their ratings to be used in marketing for the health care organizations as long as a fee is paid to the quality rating group. Many of these practices have raised concerns regarding bias in the reporting by these groups because of a lack of transparency in the rating systems. In the end, the rating system by CMS is felt by many to be the most reliable and transparent.

Summary

The measurement and reporting of health care quality have undergone dramatic change over the past two decades. This has led to a greater emphasis on quality of care delivery than in the past, and organizations, in general, are placing a greater emphasis on transparency of quality data for the public. Despite these changes, health care in the United States is not universally accepted as the standard for quality in the world, and it is unquestionably too expensive for the value it presents to patients. The chapters that follow in this book provide an extensive review of health care quality and present many ideas that can transform the US health care system. The time has come for consumers and providers of health care in our country to demand the exceptional quality and transparency that patients deserve.

References

1. Institute of Medicine (IOM). In: Kohn LT, Corrigan JM, Donaldson MS, editors. To err is human: building a safer health system. Washington, DC: National Academy Press; 2000.
2. Institute of Medicine (IOM). Crossing the quality chasm. In: Crossing the quality chasm: a new health system for the 21st century. Washington, DC: National Academy Press; 2001.
3. Berwick DM, Nolan TW, Whittington J. The triple aim: care, health, and cost. Health Aff (Millwood). 2008;27(3):759–69.
4. OECD (2020), Health spending (indicator). https://doi.org/10.1787/8643de7e-en (Accessed on 29 April 2020).
5. World Health Organization. World Health Report 2000. Geneva, 2000.
6. Verdecchia A, et al. Recent cancer survival in Europe: a 2000–02 period analysis of EUROCARE-4 data. Lancet Oncol. 2007;8(9):784–96.
7. Commonwealth Fund International Health Policy Survey of Sicker Adults. 2005.
8. Thomas EJ, Studdert DM, Newhouse JP, et al. Costs of medical injuries in Utah and Colorado. Inquiry. 1999;36:255–64.
9. Brennan TA, Leape LL, Laird L, et al. Incidence of adverse events and negligence in hospitalized patients. Results of the Harvard Medical Practice Study I. N Engl J Med. 1991;324:370–6.

Access to Affordable Health Care Coverage

5

Jessica Mantel

When people get sick or hurt, whether they receive appropriate and timely medical care depends on several factors, including the availability of health services in their community, their personal beliefs about health care, and the ability to take time-off from work. For many people, however, the most important factor is whether they can afford needed care. Given the high cost of health care in the United States, few can pay their medical bills out-of-pocket. Instead, most Americans rely on health insurance to cover all or part of the cost. Those without health insurance, however, lack the means to pay for health care. Consequently, far too often, the uninsured must postpone or forego needed services.

The underinsured—individuals whose health insurance provides inadequate financial protection—also report problems accessing health care. This is because the content of health coverage, namely, what plans will pay for, also affects access. Insurers only pay for health services that fall within the plan's scope of included health benefits and are deemed "medically necessary." In addition, enrollees may have to pay for all or a portion of a service's costs depending on the size of the plan's deductible, co-pays, and co-insurance amounts and whether the service is provided by a network provider. This means that some people with health insurance nevertheless delay or forgo needed care if their plan's coverage policies leave significant gaps in what the plan pays for.

The consequences of cutting back on needed care among the uninsured and underinsured have lasting, adverse effects on health. The uninsured are less likely to have a personal physician or other regular source of health care, which in turn makes them less likely to receive preventive and screening services such as immunizations, regular check-ups, and mammograms. As a result, illnesses and diseases that could have been averted or caught early may become serious, costly health conditions. Uninsured patients who delay or forgo other needed care also are at greater risk for

J. Mantel (✉)
University of Houston Law Center, Houston, TX, USA
e-mail: jmantel@Central.UH.EDU

© Springer Nature Switzerland AG 2020
P. V. Sreeramoju et al. (eds.), *The Patient and Health Care System: Perspectives on High-Quality Care*, https://doi.org/10.1007/978-3-030-46567-4_5

declining health and preventable medical complications. The underinsured similarly suffer poorer health and increased mortality.

While most Americans have comprehensive health insurance and do not report difficulty accessing needed care, approximately three in ten Americans report problems paying their medical bills [1]. Moreover, many people—approximately half of the population—worry about whether in the future they can afford needed care. For this reason, access to affordable, comprehensive health insurance dominates national discussions on health care. This chapter explains why some people lack access to health insurance, as well as why many people enrolled in health insurance still face challenges paying for their care. It also highlights proposals to address these issues.

Access to Affordable Health Insurance

Today, more Americans have health insurance than at any time in US history. According to the United States Census Bureau, in 2019 two-thirds of the population was insured by private plans offered through an employer or purchased directly from insurers. Government health insurance programs cover millions more. In 2019, Medicare insured over 55 million elderly and disabled individuals,[1] while in 2019 Medicaid and the Children's Health Insurance Program insured nearly 1 in 5 people, mostly low-income individuals and families.[2] Military health coverage also insures almost 5 percent of the population.[3]

The ranks of the uninsured hit historic lows following implementation of various policies put into effect under the Affordable Care Act (ACA), also known as "Obamacare." Yet despite these reforms, many Americans still lack health insurance. Over 28 million Americans, or almost 9 percent of the population, did not have health insurance at any point during 2017. While some uninsured individuals choose to forgo health insurance, most would prefer to be insured but report difficulty paying for health insurance. This section explains how the policies adopted under the ACA helped many people gain access to affordable health insurance, but left millions still uninsured.

Over half of the population has employer-based coverage, or insurance obtained through a worker's employer or a family member's employer. Employer-sponsored

---

[1] Many Medicare beneficiaries are enrolled in plans offered by private insurers. Approximately one in three Medicare beneficiaries have opted to enroll in Medicare Advantage plans offered by private insurers who contract with the federal government. In addition, some Medicare beneficiaries enroll in supplemental policies offered by private insurers (known as "Medigap") or receive supplemental coverage through retiree insurance offered by employers.

[2] Nearly all states have incorporated managed care into their Medicaid programs, with over two-thirds of Medicaid beneficiaries enrolled in Medicaid managed care plans administered by private insurers.

[3] Some individuals have two or more sources of coverage. For example, 12 million people are enrolled in both Medicare and Medicaid, and many Medicare enrollees purchase supplemental private insurance. Accordingly, the sum of the percentages of those with certain types of insurance exceeds 100 percent.

insurance is also referred to as group coverage, with small employers (those with fewer than 50 full-time employees) purchasing insurance through what is called the small group market. Typically the employer pays a portion of the plan's premium, with the employee responsible for the remaining premium. Larger employers generally pay a larger portion of the premium than smaller employers, leaving employees of smaller employers bearing a greater share of premium costs. Some workers whose employers offer health insurance elect not to enroll, as they cannot afford their share of the premium, which on average has increased at a faster rate than wage growth. For example, in 2017, nine out of ten employees who forewent employer-sponsored health insurance did so because they could not afford the employee's share of the premium [2]. Moreover, not all employers offer their employees health benefits. In 2017, 71 percent of nonelderly, uninsured workers were employed by companies that did not offer health insurance to their employees.

Although the majority of working-age adults and their families obtain health insurance through an employer, 16 percent purchase insurance directly from private insurers. The market for health insurance offered to individuals and families purchasing their own insurance is called the individual market. The individual market includes the state insurance exchanges created under the ACA, which allows consumers to compare health plans offered in their state that comply with various federal standards. The state exchanges also offer small group plans.

Historically, the individual market did not work well for many people, particularly those with existing health conditions and limited financial means. Pre-ACA, insurers evaluated an applicant's health to determine if he or she was likely to be a high consumer of medical care, a process known as "medical underwriting." Most states allowed insurers to deny coverage to high-risk individuals or families, which in 2013 happened to 18 percent of applicants [3]. Insurers likewise could refuse to renew an individual's policy at the end of the plan year if he or she became sick. Insurers also could charge high-risk individuals and their families higher premiums than other plan enrollees, premiums that often were beyond what high-risk applicants could pay. Although premiums for non-high risk individuals and families were lower, those with modest income often could not afford the premiums, opting instead to forgo health insurance.

The ACA adopted important reforms designed to promote access to affordable health insurance, regardless of age or health status. On the employer side, ACA incentivizes employers with 50 or more full-time employees to provide health insurance to their employees by penalizing those who fail to offer health benefits to at least 95 percent of their full-time workers. In addition, plans that offer dependent coverage, which includes most employer-sponsored plans, must be open to enrollees' adult children under the age of 26, regardless of whether the adult child is living with the parent, enrolled in school, or listed as a dependent on the parent's tax return.

The ACA also imposed new rules on plans offered in the individual and small group markets that make health insurance more accessible and affordable. Specifically, the ACA prohibits insurers in the individual and small group markets from denying coverage based on the applicant's health status, medical history, or medical expenses. In addition, insurers cannot cancel, discontinue, or refuse to renew coverage for reasons other than nonpayment of premiums, fraud, intentional misrepresentation of a material fact, or moving outside the plan's service area. Insurers also cannot vary premiums based on health status, medical history, use of health services, income, and gender. (Premiums, however, may vary based on age up to a maximum variation of 3:1 between older and younger adults and based on tobacco use up to a maximum variation of 1.5:1 between tobacco users and non-users.)

Those with household incomes between one to four times the federal poverty level also receive help paying their premiums for exchange plans, as long as their employer does not offer affordable, comprehensive coverage and they are ineligible for Medicare, Medicaid, or the Children's Health Insurance Program. This help takes the form of a premium tax credit, which, at the individual's election, the IRS will pay directly to the insurance company on the individual's behalf. The premium tax credit is the difference between the premium for a benchmark plan (the second-lowest "silver" plan[4] available to the individual through their state exchange) and the individual's required income contribution (ranging from approximately 2 percent of income for those at 100 percent of the federal poverty level to approximately 9.5 percent for those between 300–400 percent of the federal poverty level). For example, if the benchmark plan had an annual premium of $10,000 for a single individual, an individual earning $48,000 in 2019 would receive a maximum tax credit of $5267, or the difference between the $10,000 premium and their required income contribution of $4732. In contrast, an individual earning just above 400 percent of the federal poverty level ($48,560 for a single individual in 2019) would not get any help paying their premium.

Finally, the ACA expanded Medicaid to many low-income adults. States that have not expanded Medicaid under the ACA typically point to higher state Medicaid costs as the rationale for their not doing so, although multiple studies have found that Medicaid expansion is associated with higher economic growth and state savings from lower expenses in non-Medicaid spending.

In the 14 states that have not expanded Medicaid, however, many low-income adults fall through the cracks, as they are ineligible for Medicaid but earn too little (below the federal poverty line) to qualify for the premium tax credits that subsidize the cost of exchange plans. Consequently, states that have expanded Medicaid typically have lower uninsured rates [4].

Following full implementation of the ACA, the ranks of the uninsured among the nonelderly population declined dramatically, from over 44 million people in 2013 to just above 28 million people in 2017. Yet many people still report difficulty paying for health insurance. Over two million poor, uninsured adults fall in the so-called "coverage gap," living in states that have not expanded Medicaid to low income adults but earning too little to qualify for the premium tax credits. Among those who qualify for the premium tax credits, many do not enroll in an exchange

[4]A silver plan is an exchange plan with an actuarial value of 70 percent, which means that on average the insurer will pay 70 percent of an enrollee's health care costs for covered services.

plan. For example, only 41 percent of those eligible for the premium tax credits with incomes between 138 percent and 250 percent of the federal poverty line enroll in an exchange plan. Low enrollment rates, in part, may reflect people not realizing how much financial assistance they qualify for, but many cite cost as a continuing barrier to coverage.

However, most of the uninsured—approximately 75 percent—live in households with at least one full-time worker, with an additional 10 percent having a part-time worker in the household. As noted above, many of these individuals are not offered employer-sponsored insurance or forgo employer-sponsored health insurance because they cannot not afford the employee's share of the premium. The exchanges also may not offer working individuals and their families affordable health insurance, as the premium tax credits are unavailable to those with incomes above 400 percent of the federal poverty level. Older adults ineligible for the premium tax credits face the greatest challenge finding affordable insurance, given that plans can charge them premiums three times higher than those charged younger adults.

Looking ahead, some policy analysts expect enrollment in the individual market to decline. Beginning in 2019, individuals no longer must pay a tax penalty (known as the "individual mandate") if they lack health insurance. The Congressional Budget Office estimates that, in the absence of this tax penalty, between three and six million Americans will choose to forgo health insurance. Insurance experts believe that younger and healthier individuals are the most likely to forgo purchasing insurance, which would result in the average exchange enrollee being older and sicker than at present. The disenrollment of healthier individuals, therefore, could raise premiums for exchange plans, making them even less affordable for those ineligible for the premium tax credits.

Policymakers continue to explore options for expanding access to health insurance. In an effort to expand access and choice for individuals, in August of 2018, the Trump administration revised the regulations governing short-term health plans. Short-term plans are exempt from most of the federal consumer protection rules discussed below in Part II. For example, short-term plans do not have to cover pre-existing conditions, may exclude benefits such as maternity care and mental health treatments, and may cap annual or life-time benefits. In addition, short-term plans can reject high-risk applicants or charge them higher premiums. Because they are exempt from these rules, short-term plans have lower premiums than plans offered in the individual market. Under the Obama administration, short-term plans were limited to a 90-day period and could not be renewed, as they were intended only for those who needed health insurance for a short duration, such as individuals who were in-between jobs. The new rules, however, allow insurers to offer short-term plans for a period of up to 364 days, and they can be renewed for up to 3 years. Proponents of the new rules argue that they increase access to health insurance by providing a less expensive option for healthier individuals who do not need, and cannot afford, more comprehensive coverage. Critics, however, argue that these plans leave enrollees underinsured, exposing them to financial risk if they are injured or become sick. In addition, short-term plans may draw younger and healthier individuals out of the individual market, which could lead to higher premiums for those who remain in the individual market. The new rules are controversial and have been challenged in court.

Offering more generous premium tax credits also would expand access to affordable health insurance. As noted above, many individuals eligible for the premium tax credits do not enroll in an exchange plan, as they cannot afford the premiums even with the subsidies. To address this concern, some states offer low and moderate income individuals additional premium subsidies. For example, Massachusetts, the state with the lowest uninsured rates, offers additional premium subsidies to those with incomes below 300 percent of the federal poverty level. Congress also could pass legislation increasing the premium tax credit amounts. Congress also could eliminate the coverage gap that ensnarls those living in states that have not expanded Medicaid by abolishing the minimum income threshold for the premium tax credits. Alternatively, states that have not expanded Medicaid to all low-income adults could elect to do so.

To address the plight of workers earning too much to qualify for premium tax credits, some have proposed raising the income limit above 400 percent of the federal poverty line or eliminating it altogether. For example, a 2019 bill proposed by House Democrats would eliminate the income limit and authorize premium tax credits for anyone whose premium for their state's benchmark exchange plan exceeds 8.5 percent of their income. However, any federal legislation to expand premium tax credits would increase federal expenditures. For example, an analysis of proposed legislation that would have expanded premium tax credits to those above the 400 percent of the federal poverty level, as well as increased the premium tax credit amounts for those with lower incomes, concluded that, although the bill would extend coverage to several million people, it would cost several hundred billion dollars over 10 years.

Comprehensive Coverage

While having health insurance makes it more likely that a person can afford needed care, it does not guarantee access. Insurers do not pay for all health care desired by patients or recommended by their health care providers. Sometimes they won't pay for any of the cost; other times they will pay for only a portion of the patient's medical bill, leaving the patient responsible for paying the rest. Consequently, those with health insurance are not immune to problems with health care costs, and many report difficulty paying medical bills and delaying or forgoing needed care. This part discusses the rules governing whether a plan will pay for a patient's care and how much of the cost they will cover.

Scope of Medical Benefits

Health plans do not cover all health care expenses. Instead, they only pay for those expenses arising from a pre-defined set of conditions and services as spelled out in the plan's contract, called "covered" services or benefits. When people receive care that is not a covered service under their plan, they must pay for the service themselves. For example, if a plan does not cover mental health care, those needing mental health services must pay for these services out-of-pocket or, if unable to do so, forgo mental health care. Plans also may impose caps on specific benefits. For example, if a plan caps coverage for inpatient care at $100,000, enrollees must pay for any inpatient care costs exceeding $100,000.

Most employer-sponsored plans, particularly those offered by larger employers, cover a broad range of benefits, with few if any caps on specific benefits. Nevertheless, a 2012 study by the National Academy of Medicine found that the typical employer plan often excluded coverage of habilitation and behavioral health services, as well as chronic disease management, dental care, and vision care [5]. In addition, historically, employers with many low-wage workers, such as Walmart and McDonalds, offered their employees less generous coverage, frequently capping specific benefits such as inpatient care. Those enrolled in these so-called "skinny" plans often face significant medical bills should they require costly care.

Prior to the ACA, most plans offered in the individual market had a narrower scope of covered benefits than employer-sponsored plans. These plans commonly excluded maternity care, mental health care, and prescription drugs. Many also imposed caps on specific benefits, including annual limits on what plans would spend on covered benefits and lifetime limits on what they would spend for the duration of when an individual was enrolled (e.g., $1 million). In addition, plans offered in the individual market frequently did not cover services related to pre-existing health conditions (e.g., excluding benefits related to an insurance applicant's asthma or HIV/AIDS).

The ACA adopted important reforms designed to promote access to not only affordable insurance but also more comprehensive health insurance. Plans in the individual and small group markets must offer comprehensive coverage similar in scope to most employer plans. Specifically, all plans in the individual and small group markets must offer the "essential health benefits," which includes ambulatory services, emergency services, hospital care, maternity and newborn care, mental health and substance use disorder services, prescription drugs, rehabilitative and habilitative services and devices, laboratory services, preventive care, wellness services and chronic disease management, and pediatric services. Importantly, plans are not required to cover *all* medical care that falls within the aforementioned categories, but only the specific benefits within each category covered by the benchmark plan selected by each state (and any supplemental benefits specified by the state if the benchmark plans do not cover any services from one or more of the essential health benefits categories). The ACA requirement to cover the essential health benefits applies only to plans sold through the individual and small group markets; plans offered by large employers are free to exclude from coverage any of the essential health benefits. For example, a large employer plan may not cover physical therapy or mental health care. However, the ACA incentivizes larger employers to offer comprehensive coverage by imposing tax penalties on those who offer skinny plans. The ACA also discourages low-value employer plans by requiring large group plans to spend at least 85 percent of premium dollars on their insured's medical care, with those who fail to do so required to provide a rebate to enrollees.

In addition, with few exceptions,[5] all plans (both individual and group plans) must cover pre-existing conditions. The ACA also prohibits insurers from imposing annual and lifetime limits on the essential health benefits, meaning plans can no longer cap coverage for specific benefits or impose annual or lifetime limits on benefits that qualify as essential health benefits. Plans, however, may impose annual and lifetime limits for benefits that are not essential health benefits (e.g., dental care).

Various state and federal laws also mandate that individual and group plans cover specific benefits and provider services. For example, most states mandate coverage for autism spectrum disorders and a majority require coverage of breast reconstruction. Federal law requires plans to cover certain preventive services such as mammograms and childhood immunizations, as well as forty-eight hour hospital stays for new mothers and their infants. In addition, under the federal Mental Health Parity and Addiction Equity Act, if a health plan covers mental health conditions and substance use disorders, the coverage must be equal to the coverage of physical conditions. For example, if a plan covers unlimited physician visits or inpatient days for conditions such as diabetes, heart disease, or surgery, then it must cover unlimited physician visits and inpatient days for conditions such as depression, schizophrenia, or addiction. These parity requirements, however, only apply to plans that cover mental health conditions and substance use disorders, so they would not apply to large employer plans that elect not to cover mental health conditions and substance use disorders.

Although these various protections broaden the scope of benefits plans cover, most plans continue to exclude some benefits. For example, health insurance contracts commonly exclude adult dental care, eye exams, and glasses. Without coverage for these services, many individuals forgo dental and eye care. Other commonly excluded benefits include long-term care, hearing aids, cosmetic surgery, acupuncture, infertility treatments, weight loss surgery, routine foot care, home care, private nursing, and gender transformation procedures.

Critics of state and federal coverage mandates argue that they raise premiums, thereby contributing to higher rates of uninsured. Proponents, however, counter that mandates can lower costs, as those who forgo appropriate care that is not covered by their insurance may get sicker and require more expensive care later on. Studies of coverage mandates have found a mixed story, with some mandates contributing to higher premiums while others lower premiums.

---

[5] Grandfathered plans, or plans that existed before the ACA was passed on March 23, 2010, are exempt from some of the law's consumer protections. For example, grandfathered employer-sponsored plans may exclude coverage of pre-existing conditions for adult enrollees.

Coverage Determinations

Even if a medical service is listed as a covered benefit in a plan's contract, plans will not pay for the service if it is not "medically necessary." Although insurance contracts vary in how they define medical necessity, in general, plans will not cover health care that is not needed for the diagnosis or treatment of a patient's medical condition or does not meet accepted standards of medical practice. Most plans also will not cover health care that is experimental, that is, care of unproven benefit for the condition being diagnosed or treated. The decision on whether a service or item is medically necessary or experimental is made by the plan. So although a patient's physician may recommend a particular diagnostic test or treatment, the patient's health plan will not pay for the test or treatment if the plan determines that it is medically unnecessary or experimental.

The process by which insurers evaluate whether a service is medically necessary is called "utilization review." Insurers use varying criteria for determining whether a particular test or treatment is medically necessary given the patient's circumstances, but generally consider evidence of the test or treatment's clinical efficacy and safety and its cost relative to other medical interventions with comparable outcomes. For example, insurers will consider customary medical practice, clinical studies published in the peer-reviewed literature, clinical practice guidelines developed by respected organizations or experts, coverage policies issued by Medicare, Medicaid, and other private insurers, and whether the test or treatment has been approved by the Food and Drug Administration (FDA).

Given the complexity of many medical conditions and uncertainty in medical science, the line between medically necessary and unnecessary is often hazy. This may lead different insurers to reach contradictory conclusions about whether a specific service should be covered, even after considering the same evidence. Consequently, among patients suffering the same condition, some may have their treatment paid for by their insurer while others will be denied coverage on the grounds that the treatment is not medically necessary.

Proponents of medical necessity clauses argue that they set appropriate limits to insurers' financial exposure, as paying for care of questionable value wastes resources and raises premiums. In addition, coverage determinations protect patients from the potential clinical risks associated with inappropriate care (e.g., increased cancer risk from unnecessary CT scans). Critics, however, contend that insurers' medical necessity determinations are an unwarranted intrusion into the therapeutic setting. Moreover, the inherent indeterminacy of medical necessity judgments raises concerns that insurers might unfairly deny coverage of medically appropriate care.

Regulators have responded to these concerns by adopting various procedural protections designed to promote a fairer and timely review process. Although state laws vary, in general, health plans must tell an insured why they are denying coverage. In addition, a plan's decision to deny coverage may be appealed by the patient and/or his or her provider. First, enrollees can bring an internal appeal, a process whereby the health plan must conduct a full review of its decision to deny coverage within the time frames specified by state law. Second, to guard against internal reviewer's conflicts of interest, federal and state laws give insureds the right to seek a final level of appeal to an independent external reviewer, usually a medical expert unaffiliated with the plan. State laws also address plans' coverage criteria, such as requiring plans to review their coverage criteria annually.

These legal safeguards afford individuals some protection against arbitrary coverage denials. A 2011 report by the Government Accountability Office found that from 39 to 59 percent of internal appeals resulted in reversal of coverage denials, and from 23 to 54 percent of independent reviews overturned plans' coverage denials [6]. However, navigating the appeals process can be challenging, as it is time-consuming, emotional, and often frustrating for both patients and their providers. In addition, few sources of assistance are available to help individuals pursue an appeal other than their provider (if willing to help). These barriers to individuals exercising their appeal rights might allow some mistaken or unjust coverage denials to stand.

To address these concerns, some have called for greater transparency in insurers' medical necessity determinations. They argue that public dissemination of coverage decisions would lead to a "common law" of medical necessity, which could support more principled and consistent decision-making. In addition, collecting highly specific data from plans on their coverage practices would help regulators monitor insurers to make sure that patients are not denied coverage for medically appropriate care. For example, insurers could be required to provide data on coverage denial rates by type of condition or treatment, and the reversal rates for internal and external reviews. Such data also would allow regulators to flag coverage disparities based on patients' age, disability, income, race, English language ability, and other individual characteristics.[6] Collecting and analyzing more specific data, however, increases insurers' costs, which could result in higher premiums, and may raise privacy concerns if the data includes identifiable patient information.

Cost-Sharing

When insured individuals receive health care that is both a covered service under their plan and medically necessary, they nevertheless may have to pay for all or some of the costs. A plan's cost-sharing rules determine the portion of a covered service paid for by the enrollee. The plan's deductible is the amount the enrollee must pay for covered services before the plan will pay for care. After satisfying the deductible, the enrollee typically pays co-pays (a fixed dollar amount) or co-insurance (a percentage of the cost) for covered services, with the plan covering the remaining costs. For example, in a plan with a $2000 deductible, the enrollee must spend $2000 on covered services before the plan will begin paying for care. If after

---

[6] Currently, all exchange plans must submit annual summary data on the number of claims denied, number of internal appeals filed and overturned, and number of external appeals filed and overturned. This data, however, is not broken down by patient characteristics or conditions or the type of service, making it of limited value to regulators.

meeting the deductible the enrollee has a $25 co-pay for physician office visits, for an office visit that costs $100 the enrollee will pay $25 and the plan will pay $75.

Many individuals have higher cost-sharing obligations than they did in the past. This usually takes the form of a higher deductible, which rose by more than 200 percent between 2007 and 2017. Proponents of increased cost-sharing argue that exposing patients to the financial consequences of their health care choices will lead to more prudent medical decisions and will reduce unwarranted utilization. For example, patients may avoid expensive emergency department visits for low severity conditions than can be treated in less costly outpatient settings. Plans with high cost-sharing also are attractive to employers, as they typically have lower premiums than traditional plans. In 2018, over 43 percent of adults aged 18–64 with employer-sponsored plans were enrolled in high deductible health plans (HDHPs), as compared to 26.3 percent in 2011. Not surprisingly, as deductibles have increased, the percentage of insured individuals with high out-of-pocket spending also has grown. This change is a primary cause for the increasing number of people reporting difficulty paying for health care.

Studies show that overall, individuals enrolled in HDHPs reduce their utilization of health care services—they use fewer prescription drugs, see their physicians less often, and receive fewer diagnostic tests. Patients with high deductibles, however, do not simply reduce their utilization of low-value health care but also forgo necessary care. For example, patients with hypertension may forgo their medications, leading to poorer controlled blood pressure and increased risk of stroke, acute myocardial infarction, and renal impairment.

The ACA includes several reforms that protect individuals and families from high cost-sharing. All plans offered through the individual and small group markets must have an actuarial value of at least 60 percent, meaning that, for a typical group of enrollees, the plan is expected to pay at least 60 percent of the expenses for the essential health benefits. Similarly, the ACA incentivizes larger employers to offer comprehensive coverage by imposing tax penalties on those who fail to offer their employees plans with an actuarial value of at least 60 percent. Plans also cannot impose cost-sharing on preventive care, including recommended immunizations and screenings for colorectal and breast cancer, high blood pressure, cholesterol, depression, and alcoholism. The ACA also caps the amount enrollees in individual and group plans must pay out-of-pocket each year for the essential health benefits obtained from in-network providers (for 2019, the cap was $7900 for individuals and $15,800 for families). In addition, those with incomes between 100–250 percent of the federal poverty level who enroll in a silver plan through their state exchange are eligible for subsidies that reduce their cost-sharing obligations and lower their out-of-pocket limits. For example, an individual eligible for the cost-sharing subsidies may see their deductible reduced from $2000 to $500 and their out-of-pocket limit reduced from $7900 to $3000.

Nevertheless, many individuals still find themselves facing significant out-of-pocket costs due to high cost-sharing. In 2017, employees enrolled in high-deductible health plans had an average deductible of $2304 for single coverage and over $4400 for family coverage. Among individuals enrolling in exchange plans, in

2018, 63 percent selected a silver plan with an average deductible of $4034, and 29 percent enrolled in a bronze plan with an average deductible of $6002. Although many exchange enrollees receive subsidies that lower their deductibles and other cost-sharing, over 40 percent do not. Finally, both individual and group plans may exclude from the annual out of-pocket limit amounts paid by the enrollee for care provided by an out-of-network provider or for care that is not an essential health benefit (e.g., dental care).

Low income individuals may be especially prone to delay or forgo care due to higher cost-sharing, as many lack the financial resources to satisfy their deductibles and other cost-sharing obligations. Approximately half of families with incomes between 150 percent and 400 percent of the federal poverty line have less than $3000 in liquid assets, with low and moderate single-person households averaging even fewer assets. In addition, low-income individuals often have higher deductibles than those with higher incomes, as they are more likely to be employed at companies with higher cost-sharing requirements or enrolled in exchanges plans, which typically have higher deductibles than employer-sponsored plans.

Some health policy experts believe redesigned insurance plans could address the problem of cost-sharing, causing patients to delay or forgo appropriate care. Under "value-based insurance designs," health plans would minimize or eliminate cost-sharing for high-value services, or services shown to be highly effective and/or cost-efficient. For example, drugs that are highly effective in lowering cholesterol might have no co-pay or only a $5 co-pay. In contrast, plans would discourage low-value services by imposing higher cost-sharing on services that are less effective or not cost-efficient. While early studies of plans adopting value-based insurance designs show some improvement in patient adherence to their providers' recommendations, critics argue that broad-scale implementation would prove difficult, as many health services lack sufficient data on their clinical value.

Several bills proposed before Congress would lower exchange enrollees' cost-sharing by expanding the cost-sharing subsidies. Specifically, these bills lower cost-sharing for those already eligible by increasing the subsidy amounts and/or make more people eligible for the cost-sharing subsidies [2]. As with proposals to expand the premium tax credits, increasing the cost-sharing subsidies would increase access to care, but raise federal expenditures.

Narrow Provider Networks

Today, most health plans maintain a network of providers. Some plans require their enrolled individuals to obtain their health care from network providers, which means those seeing out-of-network providers must pay the full cost of their care. Other plans permit enrollees to see out-of-network providers, but those who do so incur higher out-of-pocket costs, as plans typically impose higher cost-sharing for out-of-network care (e.g., $4000 deductible out-of-network vs. $2000 deductible in-network, 40 percent coinsurance out-of-network vs. 20 percent coinsurance in-network). In addition, the out-of-network provider can bill the patient for the difference between their charges and what the plan is willing to pay, a practice known as "balanced billing." For example, if the provider charges $200 for a service and the plan pegs the permitted charge at $125 (called the "allowed amount"), the provider can bill the patient for the $75 difference (plus any cost-sharing obligations). Balanced billed and cost-sharing amounts paid to out-of-network providers also do not count toward the insured's out-of-pocket maximum.

Proponents of narrow networks argue that they offer several benefits. First, by selectively contracting with providers who have proven track records, plans can steer their enrollees to high quality providers. Second, plans with narrower networks have greater bargaining leverage vis-à-vis providers, as providers may accept a lower payment rate in anticipation that they will serve a larger share of a plan's enrollees. Savings from lower payment rates can be passed on to consumers in the form of lower premiums, and studies have confirmed that exchange plans with narrower networks generally have lower premiums. However, individuals who cannot afford the costs of an out-of-network provider may be unable to access needed care if there is not a qualified network provider available to them. This occurs when there are no qualified network providers within a reasonable distance from where the individual resides, qualified network providers are not accepting new patients, or no network provider is qualified to treat the individual's condition.

To address these concerns, many states have adopted network adequacy requirements for individual and small group plans. Most of these standards, however, are vague and simply require that a plan's provider network afford enrollees "reasonable access" to providers. Some states, though, impose specific quantitative standards, such as minimum provider-to-patient ratios, maximum travel times or distance to and from providers, and maximum appointment wait times. Some states also require that there be a minimum number of network providers accepting new patients. In addition, some states require plans to pay for out-of-network care when an insured lacks access to a qualified in-network provider. Unfortunately, states' enforcement of their network adequacy standards has been spotty, with many state regulators simply relying on an insurer's general attestation that its network is adequate. Moreover, few states regulate the provider networks for large group plans, relying instead on employers to police the adequacy of their plan's provider network.

To supplement state efforts, the ACA created federal oversight of the adequacy of exchange plans' provider networks. Rules adopted during the Obama administration required all exchange plans to meet maximum time and distance standards. In 2017, however, the Trump administration eliminated these specific standards, leaving it to state regulators to define network adequacy. As noted above, however, many states lack quantitative standards on network adequacy and do not closely police network adequacy. Consequently, critics fear that the Trump administration's changes will exacerbate network adequacy problems, leaving more patients with inadequate access to care.

Conclusion

Whether an individual has access to affordable health care depends on their having comprehensive health insurance. Although millions of Americans gained access to health insurance under the ACA, many still cannot afford the premiums and so remain uninsured. Moreover, among those with health insurance, countless report difficulty paying for needed care, as insurers do not pay the full cost of all health care services. Ongoing debates about health care reform will continue wrestling with how to extend health coverage while reining in costs. These discussions raise complex questions about ways to make the health care system more efficient and less costly, issues that are beyond the scope of this chapter. Yet they also focus attention on the coverage and cost trade-offs highlighted in this chapter: First, a limited scope of benefits, higher cost-sharing, aggressive utilization review policies, and narrower provider networks all lower health insurance premiums, but leave insured individuals bearing a larger proportion of their medical costs. Second, lowering individuals' premiums and cost-sharing through more generous government subsidies will expand health coverage and access to care, but require higher government health care expenditures. Striking the proper balance between these policy trade-offs is no small task, but understanding the issues will help the reader meaningfully participate in discussions about the future of US health care.

References

1. DiJulio B, et al. Data note: Americans' challenges with health care costs, 2017, March.
2. Kaiser Family Foundation. Side-by-side comparison of medicare-for-all and public plan proposals introduced in the 116th congress, 2019,May., http://files.kff.org/attachment/Table-Side-by-Side-Comparison-Medicare-for-all-Public-Plan-Proposals-116th-Congress.
3. Lueck S. Center on budget and policy priorities, eliminating federal protections for people with health conditions would mean return to dysfunctional pre-ACA individual market, 2017, May 3.
4. Kiernan JS. States with the Highest and Lowest Uninsured Rates (Oct 2019), https://wallethub.com/edu/uninsured-rates-by-state/4800/.
5. Ulmer C, et al. Essential health benefits: balancing coverage and cost, 2012.
6. Government Accountability Office. Private health insurance: data on application and coverage denials, 2011, March., https://www.gao.gov/assets/320/316699.pdf.

Bibliography

Aron-Dine A, Broaddus M. Improving ACA subsidies for low- and moderate-income consumers is key to increasing coverage, 2019, March.
Bloomberg Law, Health law & business portfolio series, health insurance & benefits, portfolio 2350: Affordable Care Act implementation: regulations, models and implications, detailed analysis, 2018.
Clayton G, et al. The Henry J. Kaiser Family Foundation, issue brief: Pre-ACA market practices provide lessons for ACA replacement approaches, 2017, Feb.

Cohen RA, et al. High-deductible health plans and financial barriers to medical care: early release of estimates from the National Health Interview Survey, 2016, U.S. DEP'T HEALTH & HUMAN SERV. 1 (June 2017), https://www.cdc.gov/nchs/data/nhis/earlyrelease/insur201708.pdf.

Congressional Budget Office. Federal subsidies for health insurance coverage for people under age 65: 2018 to 2028 (CBO, 2018, May), https://www.cbo.gov/system/files/115th-congress-2017-2018/reports/53826-healthinsurancecoverage.pdf.

Doty M, et al. The Commonwealth Fund, failure to protect: why the individual insurance market is note a viable option for most U.S. families, 2009,July.

Foutz J, et al. The uninsured: a primer: key facts about health insurance and the uninsured under the Affordable Care Act, 2017, Dec.

Giled S, et al. Effects of the affordable care act on health care access, 2017.

Hall M, Ginsberg, PB. A better approach to regulating provider network adequacy, 2017.

Hamel L, et al. The Burden of medical debt: results from the Kaiser Family Foundation/New York Times Medical Bills Survey, 2016, Jan.

Jacobi JV, et al. Health insurer market behavior after the Affordable Care Act: assessing the need for monitoring, targeted enforcement, and regulatory reform. Penn State Law Rev. 2015;120:109–79.

Kaiser Family Foundation. Employer health benefits: 2018 survey, 2018.

Kaiser Family Foundation. Key facts about the uninsured population, 2018, Dec.

Lavarreda S, et al. Underinsurance in the United States: an interaction of costs to consumers, benefit design, and access to care. Ann Rev Public Health. 2011;32:471–82.

Mantel J. How efforts to lower health care costs are putting patients and physicians on a collision course, 44 Ohio N. U. L. Rev. 371, 2018.

Pear R. 'Short term' health insurance? up to 3 years under New Trump Policy, New York Times, 2018, Aug 1.

Pollitz K, Cox C. Medical debt among people with health insurance, 2014, Jan.

United States Census Bureau, Health insurance coverage in the United States: 2017, 2018, Sept.

U.S. Department of Health and Human Services, Office of Inspector General. Medicare advantage appeal outcomes and audit findings raise concerns about service and payment denials, 2018., https://oig.hhs.gov/oei/reports/oei-09-16-00410.pdf.

Access to Affordable Health Care: Health Care Executive Perspective

6

John Jay Shannon

Introduction

In her chapter on Access to Affordable Health Care Coverage, Prof. Jessica Mantel nicely laid out the complexities and expenses of obtaining health care insurance and the challenges for individuals inherent in our complex patchwork of private and governmental insurance programs. In this chapter, I will describe challenges for providers, especially hospitals and physicians, working within the current insurance environment. This chapter will focus on governmental insurance products, as growth in those plans has driven the recent historical drop in uninsured rates in this country (see Fig. 6.1), and policy regarding Medicare payments and strategies (such as bundled payments and Value-Based Purchasing) in particular drives strategies and payments from commercial insurers. The cost of health care and improving insurance coverage for more Americans is also the focus of an ongoing national debate.

Health care expenditures in the United States are the highest in the world. According to the Centers for Medicare and Medicaid Services, US health care spending in 2018 reached $3.6 trillion. That is $11,172 *per person*, and 17.7% of the nation's Gross Domestic Product. That same year, the median US household income was $63,179 (US Census Bureau). On a per capita basis, health spending has increased over 30-fold in the last four decades, from $355 per person in 1970 to $10,739 in 2017. In constant 2017 Dollars, the increase was almost sixfold from $1797 in 1970 to $10,739 in 2017. Given the high costs of health care, most cannot pay out of-pocket for care.

Today, fully one-third of all health expenditures is to hospitals. Payments to physician and other clinical professionals follow at 20%. From the perspective of those providing the services, those expenditures were reimbursed by private health insurance (34%), Medicare (21%), Medicaid (16%) and the patient's own wallet (10%) [1].

J. J. Shannon (✉)
Department of Medicine, Cook County Health, Chicago, IL, USA
e-mail: jjshannon@cookcountyhhs.org

© Springer Nature Switzerland AG 2020
P. V. Sreeramoju et al. (eds.), *The Patient and Health Care System: Perspectives on High-Quality Care*, https://doi.org/10.1007/978-3-030-46567-4_6

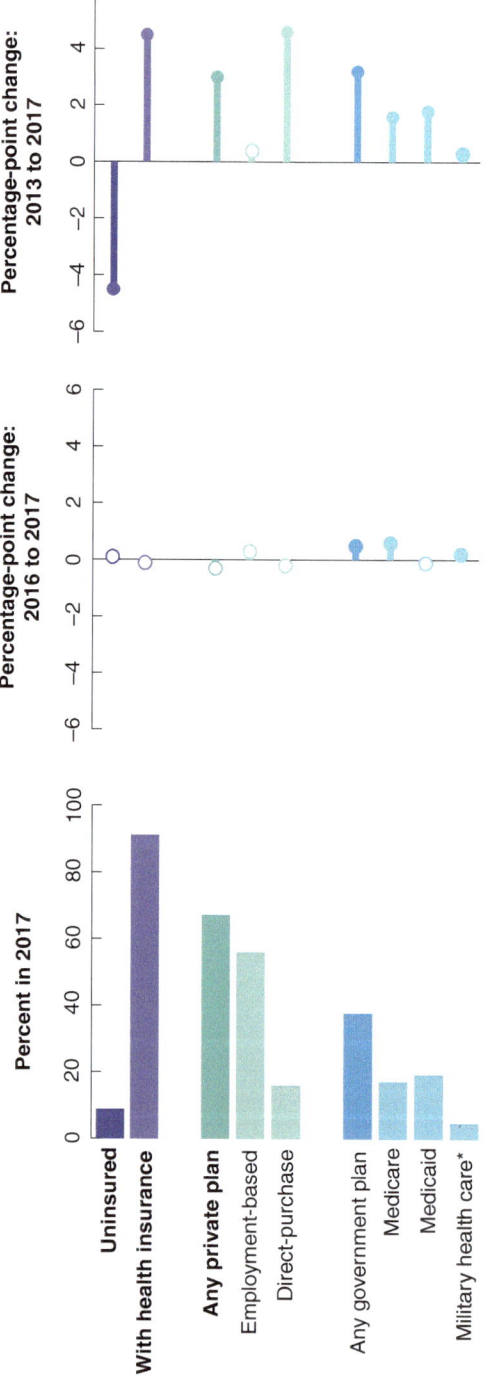

72   J. J. Shannon

Fig. 6.1 Percentage of people by type of health insurance coverage and change from 2013 to 2017 (population as of March of the following year). ○ Changes between the estimates are not statistically different from zero at the 90% confidence level. * Military health care includes TRICARE and CHAMPVA (Civilian Health and Medical Program of the Department of Veterans Affairs), as well as care provided by the Department of Veterans Affairs and the military. Note: For information on confidentiality protection, sampling error, nonsampling error, and definitions in the current population survey, see www2.census.gov/programs-surveys/cps/techdocs/cpsmar18.pdf. (Source: US Census Bureau, Current Population Survey, 2014, 2017, and 2018 Annual Social and Economic Supplements)

Government-sponsored Health Programs

Medicaid is a joint federal/state insurance program for low-income individuals, originating with an expansion of the Social Security Act in 1965 along with the introduction of Medicare. Medicaid is administered by state agencies, but funding comes from a combination of state general revenue, or health provider "taxes" that then draw down federal dollars (the Federal Medical Assistance Percentages or "FMAP", which in 2020 contributed 50–73% of total state Medicaid expenditures). Prior to the ACA, few low-income adults were eligible for Medicaid. Under the ACA, states may expand Medicaid coverage to adults with incomes at or below 138% of the federal poverty line and, as of December 2019, 36 states and the District of Columbia have done so. As of spring 2019, Medicaid enrollment had grown from pre-ACA levels by 15 million [2].

The effect of Medicaid coverage on access to care for individuals has been mixed, with varying results on wait times and appointment availability ("Coverage does not equal access") [3].

A 2018 study by the Government Accountability Office found that low-income individuals frequently forgo care, do not see physicians, and skip prescription doses in states that have not expanded Medicaid [4]. States that have not expanded Medicaid under the ACA typically point to the increasing costs associated with covering the state share for newly-insured individuals. On the other hand, expansion has been associated in multiple studies with economic growth and state savings from reduction in expenses in other areas.

The importance of Medicaid as coverage for low-income populations and a revenue source for health care providers caring for them cannot be overstated. Today, Medicaid and the related Children's Health Insurance Program (CHIP) are the payer for care for more than 70 million Americans, roughly one in five. Similarly, in Illinois, Medicaid is the insurance for roughly 20% of the state population, but it provides critical insurance for roughly one-half the children in the state, one-half of the deliveries in the state, and it is by far the single largest provider of payment for individuals in long-term care environments. At the same time, Illinois has the lowest annual per-enrollee spend of 50 states (at approximately $5000/member/year, significantly behind the national Medicaid spend of $8000/enrollee/year), and this low spend means often very low Medicaid rates, which often leads to providers refusing to care for or limiting their panel size for Medicaid-insured individuals, and for hospitals and health systems to limit the access of Medicaid-insured individuals in overt (refusing to contract with Medicaid health plans) and subtle (different queues for different payers) ways.

Medicaid payments to hospitals are theoretically matched to costs of care; the Kaiser Family Foundation estimate overall Medicaid payment to hospitals range from 90% to 107%, but supplemental Medicaid payments may increase reimbursement above costs. On the other hand, using different methodologies, the American Hospital Association estimates hospitals are only reimbursed 87 cents on the dollar of care for Medicaid and Medicare enrollees. Denials from Medicaid managed care plans are for many hospitals significantly higher than for any insurance payer.

Medicare is a critical insurance program for individuals over 65 years of age, with significant disabilities, or with end stage renal disease. Created as an expansion of the Social Security Act in 1965, it is funded by contributions from direct payroll deductions of working individuals, supplemented by employer contributions; federal income tax revenues, and premiums (for parts B and D), and co-pays from members. Today, Medicare insures almost 60 million Americans. Enrollees can elect for coverage of hospital care, physician and outpatient charges, and drug benefits. Enrollment is managed by the Social Security Administration, and premiums are typically deducted monthly from an enrollee's Social Security income. Program strategies and rules are determined by the Centers for Medicare and Medicaid Services. There is no cap on out-of-pocket expenses, so most enrollees choose to carry additional ("Medigap") insurance or enroll in a managed Medicare program with caps (Medicare Advantage). If a beneficiary has very low income, they may also qualify for Medicaid, so-called "dual-eligible" status. In this arrangement, Medicaid can pay expenses ordinarily paid by a Medicare beneficiary, including deductibles, copays, premiums, some drug and care coordination costs.

Prior to the passage of Medicare, some 40% of American seniors was uninsured, so Medicare has provided peace of mind for American seniors—but program funding is tenuous, given demographic shifts (an increasing number of beneficiaries and a decreasing number of young workers paying into the program) and health care inflation. With increasing health care costs overall, it is predicted that an ever-increasing proportion of Social Security income will be spent by retirees on out-of-pocket health care costs. A recent study of seriously ill Medicare enrollees found that more than half were challenged financially with out-of-pocket expenses [5].

Marketplace Plans

The previous chapter described how the ACA supports individuals with incomes from one to four times the federal poverty level to buy health insurance on insurance exchanges, so called "marketplace" plans. A significant rationale for expansion of health insurance coverage under the Obama administration's Patient Protection and Affordable Care Act (ACA) was the fundamental insurance concept of "risk pools": the more subscribers to an insurance product, the greater the likelihood of premium-paying members who would not make claims on the insurance product. The so-called Individual Mandate in the ACA penalized individuals eligible for a health insurance plan if they did not subscribe. While this was a modest penalty, it was reversed by the Tax Cuts and Jobs Act of 2018, which made the mandate meaningless by zeroing out the penalty. While it is too early to estimate the impact this repeal will have on insurance-seeking behavior, the Congressional Budget Office estimates some 3–6 million Americans will choose to forgo health insurance in the early years of repeal [6]. Insurance experience would suggest that those most likely to forgo purchasing insurance will be those who are healthiest ("young invincibles") or those with the least disposable income, thus disrupting the model of distributing insurance pool risk.

Marketplace plans may be associated with significant annual deductibles (in the thousands of dollars), so oftentimes providers are faced with an individual who is technically insured, but who is unable to pay the "first dollars" of health care coverage called for in their deductible—and this portion of medical billing often falls into uncollectable Bad Debt (vide infra).

EMTALA

As a last resort for the uninsured or underinsured, the Emergency Medical Treatment and Labor Act (EMTALA) is a federal law passed in 1986 that requires hospitals to treat and stabilize anyone presenting to an emergency department with an emergency medical condition, regardless of insurance status or ability to pay. While EMTALA has significantly decreased the practice of private hospitals "dumping" on public safety net hospitals, challenges persist. First, EMTALA does not come with federal funding for care; thus, expenses related to EMTALA for an uninsured individual typically fall to a hospital's uncompensated care costs as Bad Debt. Second, EMTALA does not apply to an individual that does not need acute care. Thus, a person may present uninsured to a hospital emergency room in crisis that requires acute treatment, such as a gastrointestinal hemorrhage that turns out to be due to an underlying colonic neoplasm, or with a complication of untreated diabetes mellitus or hypertension. Once the acute circumstance is addressed and the patient is stabilized, there is no obligation for that hospital or more importantly, its physicians, to continue to treat that uninsured individual. Therefore, analysis of the payor mix of a hospital often shows a higher proportion of Medicaid or no insurance on the inpatient side than on the outpatient profile.

Challenges to Providers

Uncompensated Care

Uncompensated care for hospitals is typically characterized as the sum of Charity Care and Bad Debt. These terms have formal definitions for accounting purposes, but in essence Charity Care is the cost associated with caring for those individuals who meet a hospital's Charity Care program (debt is forgiven), while Bad Debt refers to costs that cannot be recovered after providing services to an individual with insurance or who claims Self Pay status (debt cannot be collected). Since the ACA has been in effect, the national trend has been falling Charity Care (more people insured overall) and rising Bad Debt (combination of poor collections from individuals with incomes above a hospital's charity care program, those unable to pay a health plan deductible or co-pay, health insurer denials). Analyses suggest that expenses provided to individuals unable to meet their deductible payments are driving these trends. In 2017, US hospitals provided an estimated $38.4 billion in uncompensated care (Source: AHA Annual Survey Data, 1995–2017). Smaller hospitals, government-controlled hospitals, and hospitals with low proportions of Medicare patients have the highest ratios of bad debt expense as a percentage of revenue.

Charity Care

To maintain their status as charitable organizations protected from property and sales taxes, not-for-profit hospitals and systems must demonstrate to the Internal Revenue Service the dollar value of community benefit they provide, and that they inform individuals struggling to pay their bills financial assistance policies in place. There has been an ongoing battle between federal and some state legislators and the hospital industry about how those conditions are being met. Actual dollars expended on charity care are usually much smaller than community benefits claimed by hospitals on their reports to the IRS (Schedule H of IRS form 990).

The Uninsured

While the ACA has brought the largest drop in the uninsured in modern history, there is still a significant number of Americans without insurance. Who are the uninsured? Working-age adults made up a much larger share of the uninsured population than any other age group. In fact, most uninsured people (84.6%) were 19–64-year-olds. Many have less than a high school education and lower income. About 4 in 10 uninsured people were non-Hispanic white, while nearly 6 in 10 people in the United States were non-Hispanic white. The uninsured were disproportionately concentrated in the South, due to slower uptake of the Affordable Care Act in the southern states (See Fig. 6.2).

The uninsured population was also disproportionately more likely to live in poverty. About 1 in 3 uninsured workers were in service occupations, compared with about 1 in 5 workers in the United States overall (Fig. 6.3).

"Churn"

Churn refers to the disruption and variability in health care coverage that occurs when people lose eligibility for one coverage and may go for a period without coverage. For example, Medicaid is determined by current monthly income, and beneficiaries may fall off coverage if they see a temporary pay increase, only to need Medicaid coverage again when income falls. During a time of income increase, the individual may qualify for a marketplace option, but open enrollment may be closed, or an individual may take their chances and go "naked", hoping for no health crises. No doubt the personal impetus to obtain coverage has lessened since the Individual Mandate penalty was reduced to zero. Perhaps predictably based on the aforementioned concept of risk pools, it has been estimated that the de facto repeal of the Individual Mandate is responsible for an increase in marketplace premiums [7]. These phenomena place administrative burdens on states and Medicaid-managed

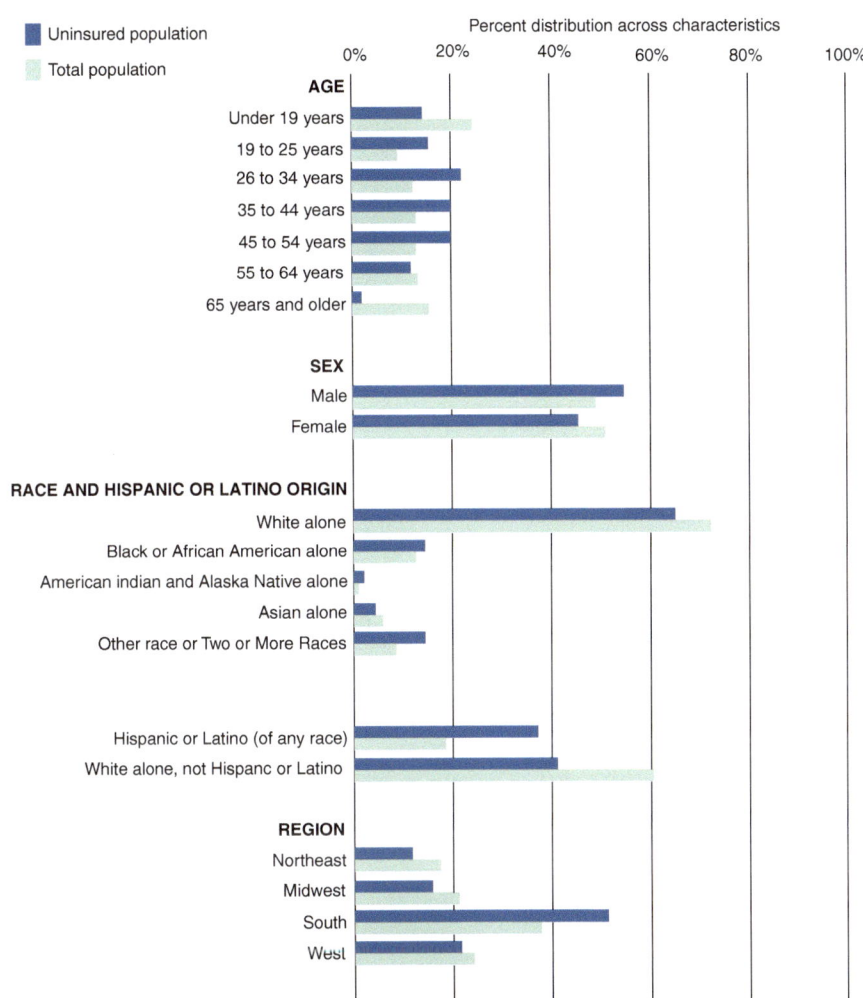

Fig. 6.2 Demographic characteristics of the uninsured and total populations: 2017. Note: Estimates are for the civilian noninstitutionalized population. For more information on the American Community Survey, see www.cenus.gov/progams-surveys/acs/. (Source: US Census Bureau 2017 American Community Survey 1-Year Estimates)

care plans, but also cause significant problems for patients seeking care and for providers hoping to be reimbursed for care they give.

Managed Care

Policies driven by cost management and pursuit of better value for health care expenditures have driven trends for both Medicaid and Medicare to increasingly be structured as managed care plans administered by private insurance companies. The

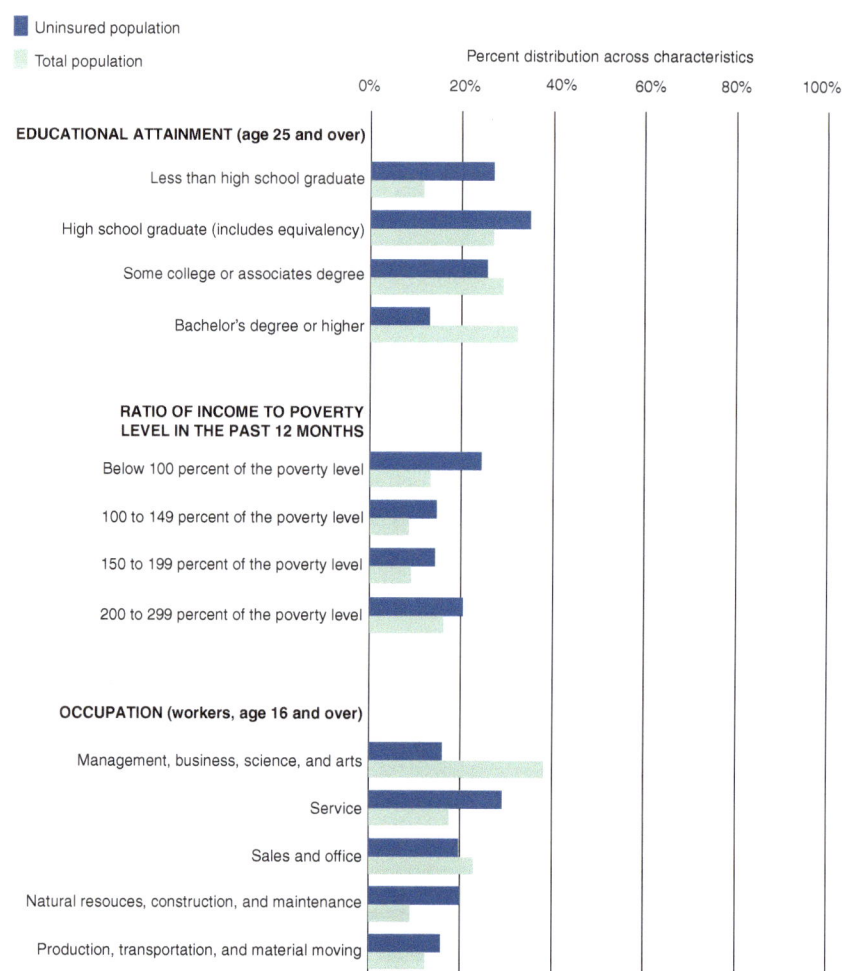

Fig. 6.3 Socio-economic characteristics of the uninsured and total population: 2017. Note: Estimates are for the civilian noninstitutionalized population. (Source: US Census Bureau 2017 American Community Survey 1-Year Estimates)

precept driving managed care is that placing an insurance company at risk for all expenses related to a beneficiary's care will drive risk assessment of members, utilization of only evidence-based care within a network of high-quality providers, and care coordination for high-risk members or conditions, and thus drive down costs. Today, about one-third of Medicare enrollees is in a Medicare Advantage plan, and Medicaid beneficiaries in 39 states are in a managed Medicaid plan.

For hospitals and physician practices, the move away from fee-for-service models for these governmental payers has meant an increase in administrative burden (e.g., obtaining pre-authorization before expensive interventions, "credentialing" of providers within multiple contracted plans), and demand for technology and staff to drive collections from multiple payers [8]. Certainly, doctors and hospitals see increased claims denials in the new managed care environment, and this is particularly acute when the payer is a Medicaid managed care organization [9, 10]. Certainly, this has led to an explosive growth in personnel necessary for revenue cycle performance, from coders, to denials management specialists, to physician advisors. Whether these administrative challenges, which lead ultimately to growing expenses for administration expenses rather than clinical expenditures, will be offset by improved health outcomes related to the benefits of care coordination remain to be seen.

Moving Forward

A recent study highlights substantial administrative expenses incurred by both providers and insurers in the United States, driven by the administrative burden associated with a multiple-payer system, and the transition of Medicare and Medicaid to a managed care-dominant format [11].

Given the costs of health care and the impact it is having on the rest of the economy, certain academics say it's clear that two things need to happen in the United States: Everyone needs to be in the health system (via insurance or a government-run system like Medicare-for-all), and cost control strategies must be developed and implemented. These strategies may include eliminating expenditures on unproven or unnecessary or repeated/wasted interventions, having price caps on drugs, allowing governmental payors more leeway when bargaining with drug manufacturers on prices, and increasing government stringency regarding decisions to cover some procedures and therapies. It is worth noting that as slim as margins may be, health care systems and insurers continue to show very significant profits, and physicians are among the highest paid professionals in the country, so complaints of low reimbursement are likely to fall on deaf ears of the general public and business leaders.

References

1. https://www.cms.gov/Research-Statistics-Data-and-Systems/Statistics-Trends-and-Reports/NationalHealthExpendData/NationalHealthAccountsHistorical. Accessed 01/11/2020.
2. https://www.medicaid.gov/medicaid/program-information/medicaid-and-chip-enrollment-data/report-highlights/index.html.
3. Antonisse L, Garfield R, Rudowitz R, Guth M. The Effects of Medicaid Expansion under the ACA: Updated Findings from a Literature Review. Washington, DC: Kaiser Family Foundation; 2019.
4. Access to Health Care for Low-Income Adults in States with and without Expanded Eligibility. U.S. Government Accountability Office. GAO-18-607. Sepember 13, 2018. https://www.gao.gov/assets/700/694489.pdf.
5. Kyle MA, Blendon RJ, Benson JM, Abrams MK, Schneider EC. Financial hardships of Medicare beneficiaries with serious illness. Health Aff (Millwood). 2019. https://doi.org/10.1377/HLTHAFF.2019.00362.

6. Congressional Budget Office. Federal subsidies for health insurance coverage for people under age 65: 2018 to 2028. CBO; 2018. https://www.cbo.gov/system/files/115th-congress-2017-2018/reports/53826-healthinsurancecoverage.pdf.
7. Kamal R, Cox C, Fehr R, Ramirez M, Horstman K, Levitt L. How repeal of the individual mandate and expansion of loosely regulated plans are affecting 2019 premiums. Kaiser Family Foundation Issue Brief, October 26, 2018. http://files.kff.org/attachment/Issue-Brief-How-Repeal-of-the-Individual-Mandate-and-Expansion-of-Loosely-Regulated-Plans-are-Affecting-2019-Premiums.
8. Hinton E, Rudowitz R, Diaz M, Singer N. 10 things to know about Medicaid managed care. Kaiser Family Foundation Issue Brief, December 16, 2019. http://files.kff.org/attachment/Issue-Brief-10-Things-to-Know-about-Medicaid-Managed-Care.
9. Medicare Advantage appeal outcomes and audit findings raise concerns about service and payment denials. U.S. Department of Health and Human Services. Office of the Inspector General. (OEI-09-16-00410). September 25, 2018. https://oig.hhs.gov/oei/reports/oei-09-16-00410.asp.
10. Gottlieb JD, Shapiro AH, Dunn A. The complexity of billing and paying for physician care. Health Aff (Millwood). 2018. https://doi.org/10.1377/hlthaff.2017.1325.
11. Himmelstein DU, Campbell T, Woolhandler S. Health care administrative costs in the United States and Canada, 2017. Ann Intern Med. 2020. https://doi.org/10.7326/M19-2818.

Part III

Quality of Care in Greater Detail

Health and Health Care Disparities: The Next Frontier in Population Health?

7

Keith Kosel and Donna Persaud

Introduction

Definition

Health care is continuously evolving, moving slowly from an industry dominated by physicians and hospitals to one that increasingly places the patient at the center of the matrix, and from a focus on inpatient care to ambulatory and virtual care, and from a focus on care of the individual patient to the health of large populations. One aspect of this industry metamorphosis has, until fairly recently, been conspicuously absent—attention to health inequities and the resulting health disparities. According to the National Institutes of Health (NIH), health disparities are differences that exist among specific population groups in the United States in the attainment of full health potential, and that can be measured by incidence, prevalence, mortality, and other adverse health conditions [1]—in other words, the higher burden of illness, injury, disability, or mortality. Health disparities often stem from health inequities, which are defined as systematic differences in the health of groups and communities occupying unequal positions in society that are unjust and avoidable [2]. According to the World Health Organization, the social determinants of health (SDOH)—the "upstream" conditions in which persons are born, grow, live, work, and age—are mostly responsible for health inequities. It is these health inequities and resulting health disparities, among other factors, that contribute to the relatively low standing of the United States in positive health outcomes and overall health status compared to its industrialized peers, despite the fact that the United States outspends all other nations [3]. In contrast to health disparities, health care disparities typically refer to differences between groups

K. Kosel
Population Health Group, Parkland Center for Clinical Innovation, Dallas, TX, USA

D. Persaud (✉)
Population Health, Parkland Health & Hospital System, Dallas, TX, USA
e-mail: Donna.Persaud@phhs.org

in "downstream" conditions, such as health insurance coverage, access to and use of care, and quality of care. In part because the terms are often used interchangeably and incorrectly, the interface between the two becomes a gray-zone, where cause and effect become difficult to untangle. For the purposes of this chapter, we focus on both health and health care disparities, but bring in numerous examples of health inequities that exist today and how we can bridge the current socioeconomic and infrastructural gaps that give rise to health and health care disparities.

While the term disparities often refers to differences between racial or ethnic groups, it increasingly encompasses many other dimensions, such as age, gender, sexual orientation, and socioeconomic position [4]. It is therefore no surprise that the issue of health disparities conjures up all sorts of emotional touchstones for people, including providers, administrators, and policymakers. In the United States, we continue to struggle with the philosophical question of whether health and health care are rights or privileges. Many argue this duality of ideas underlies many of the reasons for disparities in health care. In this chapter, we will explore many of the health care disparities that exist today, the reasons for the gaps, and what is being done to reduce or eliminate these differences.

Background

The burden of illness, premature death, and disability disproportionately affects certain populations. While disparities in health have existed for centuries, only recently has the subject become the focus of targeted studies to quantify and describe the nature, scope, and impact of these differences. The 1985 United States Department of Health and Human Services (HHS) *Secretary's Taskforce Report on Black and Minority Health* was the first signal of serious governmental concern with health disparities [5]. In 2003, the National Academy of Medicine (NAM) report, *Unequal Treatment: Confronting Racial and Ethnic Disparities in Health Care,* clearly documented the health care system's under-treatment and poor treatment of specific groups in American society [6]. In 2009, data from the REACH U.S. Risk Factor Survey of some thirty US communities indicated that residents in mostly minority communities continue to have lower socioeconomic status, greater barriers to accessing health care, and greater risk and burden of disease compared to the general population living in the same geographical area [7]. Progress in addressing disparities has been painfully slow, as noted by the 2012 and 2013 National Health Care Disparities Reports. Of those disparities involving access to care, none showed any measurable improvement since they were first identified some 10 years earlier [8].

Impact

Disparities in health care access and quality can result in substantial direct and indirect costs to society. A 2009 study estimated that eliminating health disparities for minorities during the period 2003 to 2006 would have reduced direct medical care expenses by $229.4 billion and indirect costs associated with chronic illness and premature death by approximately $1 trillion [9]. A more recent study in 2018 estimated that disparities account for approximately $93 billion in excess medical costs and $42 billion in lost productivity every year [10]. The aggregate impact of health care disparities often obscures the real cost at the patient and family levels. Across nearly all categories, minority populations had higher: (1) drug-induced deaths; (2) homicide rates; (3) prevalence of asthma, periodontitis, stroke, and coronary artery disease; (4) preventable hospitalizations; and (5) work-related deaths than their non-minority counterparts [11].

Responses to the Problem

While the challenge of addressing health care disparities appears daunting, much more work is occurring to better understand the causes of disparities and the policies and practices that allow health care disparities to exist. This work largely began with the landmark Heckler Report [5] and the first major legislation aimed at reducing disparities—the Affordable Care Act of 2011 (ACA) and its accompanying expansion of Medicaid. Recent work by the Centers for Disease Control and Prevention (CDC), the Agency for Health Care Research and Quality (AHRQ), and many other federal, state, and local agencies has also put a face on health care disparities and this work has begun the process of slowly narrowing the gap between disparate populations in the United States. The remainder of this chapter examines some of the underlying issues, the gaps, and innovative solutions, including perspectives from several key stakeholder groups.

Current State, Gaps, and Promising Solutions

Present State

According to Healthy People 2010, in addition to race and ethnicity, a host of other factors, from economic stability, education, and physical environment to community and social context, shape an individual's ability to achieve optimal health [12]. Health and health care disparities are commonly viewed through the prism of race and ethnicity, but as pointed out in the subsequently updated Healthy People 2020, they occur across a broad range of dimensions from socioeconomic status to language, geography, and citizenship status. Efforts to understand and address health care disparities have focused on designated priority populations who historically have been vulnerable to health care inequities, including people of color, low-income groups, women, older adults, individuals with disabilities, and individuals living in rural areas. It is important to recognize that these groups are not mutually exclusive and often interact in important and not-so-obvious ways. Disparities also occur within subgroups of populations.

For example, binge drinking is more common among persons aged 18–34 years, men, non-Hispanic Whites, and persons with higher household incomes [11].

Today, many groups face substantial disparities in access to and utilization of care. Despite some progress, racial and ethnic disparities are arguably the most apparent and entrenched inequities and are important for a number of reasons. As a nation, we possess an abundance of health care facilities, cutting-edge technologies, and pharmacotherapeutics that are the envy of the world, but that are not accessible, for many reasons, to all segments of the population. As a result, inadequate, inaccessible, and/or poor medical care further exacerbates poor health status for many of our citizens, while driving up the cost of care for everyone. For example, people of color generally face more access barriers and utilize less care than Whites. Among nonelderly adults, Hispanics, Blacks, American Indians, and Alaska Natives are more likely than Whites to go without needed care. Further, nonelderly Black and Hispanic adults are less likely than their White counterparts to have a usual source of care or to have had a health or dental visit in the previous year. Low-income individuals also experience more barriers to care and generally receive poorer quality care than high-income individuals [13].

Data over the past 30–40 years is compelling—health and disease states, including mental and behavioral conditions, are not evenly distributed among all groups comprising the US populace. Some populations are at higher risk for health conditions and experience poorer health outcomes compared to other populations or subpopulations. Blacks, American Indians, and Alaska Natives are more likely than Whites to be afflicted with a range of chronic health conditions, including asthma, diabetes, and heart disease [14]. Health disparities are particularly evident around AIDS and HIV diagnoses and death rates, with Blacks experiencing over eight to ten times higher rates of HIV and AIDS diagnoses than Whites [14]. Similar disparities are seen in other areas as well. Infant mortality for Black babies is nearly 2.5 times higher than for White babies, while life expectancy for Black men is nearly a decade shorter than their White counterparts. Diabetes rates are 30% higher among Native Americans and Hispanics than among Whites, while death rates due to heart disease, stroke, and certain types of cancers (breast and prostate) remain much higher in Black populations [15]. Interestingly, while the prevalence of some mental /behavioral conditions are lower among minority groups, the disability resulting from such conditions is disproportionately high. For example, rates of depression are lower among Blacks (24.6%) and Hispanics (19.6%) than Whites (34.7%), but depression in Blacks and Hispanics is more persistent [16].

One area that has received extensive study is the "unequal treatment" afforded to minorities, particularly in the area of cardiovascular care. A joint study by the American College of Cardiology and the Kaiser Family Foundation affirmed that there was credible evidence that African Americans were less likely than Whites to receive diagnostic and revascularization procedures (i.e., cardiac catheterization and angioplasty) and thrombolytic therapy, even when patient clinical characteristics were similar [17]. These disparities of care were even evident in the Veterans Affairs health care system [18].

Data from numerous studies suggest that, for many Americans, a major contributor to the problem of health disparities is the cost of, and access to, required medical care; clear discrepancies exist in the rates of health insurance coverage among Black and Hispanic populations. As would be expected, the results of being uninsured are considerable and include use of fewer preventative services, poorer health outcomes, higher mortality and disability rates, and advanced stages of illness when first diagnosed. The uninsured tend to be disproportionately poor, young, and from racial and/or ethnic minority groups.

Efforts to Close the Gaps

Proponents of the ACA hoped that the law's major insurance-expansion coverage provisions and associated system reforms would begin to narrow the disparities gap in health care for many groups facing such disparities. The ACA's broadened coverage and increased funding for community health centers was designed to improve access, while other ACA provisions mandated improved quality of care. Various ACA provisions focused specifically on reducing disparities through the creation of the Office of Minority Health within HHS. The ACA also included funding for prevention and public health initiatives and permanently reauthorized the Indian Health Care Improvement Reauthorization Extension Act of 2009.

Additionally, in 2011, HHS developed The Disparities Action Plan for eliminating racial and ethnic health disparities in the United States by setting out a series of priorities, strategies, actions, and goals to achieve a vision of "a nation free of disparities in health and health care." [19]. Two years later, HHS updated the national standards for Culturally and Linguistically Appropriate Services (CLAS), which seek to help reduce disparities and achieve health equity by ensuring that people receive care in a culturally and linguistically appropriate manner.

Given all these changes, the obvious question is "have these efforts made a difference in closing the disparities gap?" In a 2017 Commonwealth Fund study [20], the authors found that the ACA has had a material effect on narrowing long-standing disparities between White and minority populations. Specifically, the study found:

- The rates of uninsured Black and Hispanic adults declined by 9 and 12 percentage points respectively; disparities in uninsured areas decreased.
- Fewer adults skipped needed care (doctor's visits) because of costs; this translated into 2.4 million more Black and Hispanic adults, 18 years and older, seeking care than previously would have.
- Fewer adults lacked a usual source of care; that is, someone considered a personal doctor or health care provider.
- For nonelderly minority adults living in states with expanded Medicaid coverage, the number of uninsured dropped among all segments of the population, but the drop was steepest for Blacks (4 percentage points), Asians (4 percentage points), and Hispanics (3 percentage points), thus narrowing the gap between their White counterparts.

While continued efforts to enroll eligible minority individuals into coverage could contribute to further reductions in the number of uninsured and a further narrowing of the disparities gap, recent reductions in outreach and enrollment funding (specifically federal marketplace Navigators) may limit further gains. Because reductions or limits in Medicaid funding disproportionately affect people of color and low-income individuals, a proposal to reduce Medicaid funding itself or to implement new, more restrictive policy requirements would likely widen coverage disparities by race, ethnicity, and income.

Perspectives on Disparities in Health and Health Care

Physicians

As one would assume, physicians are at the "sharp end of the spear" when one considers health and health care disparities and potential solutions. Unfortunately, despite some early efforts at awareness and change, the physician community has been initially slow to take up the mantle of disparities. Not until the 2002 NAM Report, *Unequal Treatment: Confronting Racial and Ethnic Disparities in Health Care* [6] did the physician community take a collective stand to raise awareness and effect change. The NAM report found that five factors contribute to the gaps seen in US health and health care disparities. Two of their findings related directly to physicians: (1) Bias, stereotyping, prejudice, and clinical uncertainty contribute to disparities; and (2) Evidence indicates that minority patients are more likely to refuse treatment than White patients. These findings became the genesis for many subsequent studies in the literature dealing with provider bias and its impact on care.

It is widely reported in the literature that the attitudes and behavior of health care providers, especially physicians, have been cited as one of the many factors that contribute to health and health care disparities. Implicit attitudes—those that exist outside of conscious awareness—are particularly problematic. A major 2015 study of implicit bias and its effect on health care outcomes found that most health care providers appear to have implicit bias in terms of positive attitudes toward White patients and negative attitudes toward people of color [21]. The study also showed that compared to White patients, people of color were also less satisfied with their interactions with health care providers. Numerous other studies have identified a host of physician behaviors negatively impacting care of minorities, such as spending less time with patients, recommending different treatment options for minorities than their White counterparts, and approaching minority patients with a dominant and condescending tone.

While many of these physician-centric barriers still exist, organizations like the American Medical Association (AMA) and prestigious medical centers like the Cleveland Clinic are taking steps to raise awareness of the importance of eliminating health and health care disparities for both patients and the economy. The AMA has elevated the work of its Commission to End Health Care Disparities first formed in 2007 and has developed numerous tools and provider resources to help address disparities. The Commission is also determining better ways to collect and use patient-level data on race, ethnicity, preferred language, and gender status and is working with the nation's colleges and universities to help create a diversified health care workforce that is more likely to serve minority and underserved populations.

Nurses

The goal of eliminating health disparities and ultimately achieving health equity will not be realized without the active support of nurses and the nursing profession. Nurses have long played a central role in caring for patients and establishing relationships with both patients and their families. Historically, nurses provided care to the most in need and the most unfortunate in society. They have advocated for the poor and the suffering with little distinction as to one's skin color. As the nursing profession has gradually become more ruled by the scientific model and technology, some of these aspects of caring and advocacy have been replaced by a focus on administrative roles and other non-patient-facing priorities, such as education, research, and workforce development. While the focus of reducing disparities has been on the individual physician, the focus of reducing disparities in nursing has targeted the broader infrastructure. As noted in a 2014 article, the nursing profession will be challenged to recruit and retain a culturally diverse workforce that mirrors the nation's changing demographics against a backdrop of low minority enrollment in our nation's nursing schools [22]. Efforts to diversify the nursing workforce should include a measurable strategic plan to recruit and retain racial/ethnic minority individuals in nursing schools, increase the number of minority faculty teaching in these programs, and increase the number of nurses in health care leadership positions. The reduction of health disparities will not be fully realized without successfully addressing the underrepresentation of minority nurses in the field and in leadership in our health care institutions.

Public Health

Over the past several decades, researchers and policymakers have developed a number of frameworks to conceptualize factors influencing health care access as it relates to disparities. While most of the frameworks focus on individual-level factors, such as demographics, personal health beliefs, health insurance status, etc., more recent studies point to the importance of community-level factors in the genesis of the gaps seen between various populations. As demonstrated by the CDC's foundational work in 2011 around disparities in health and health care, public health agencies and public health personnel represent an important conduit to address disparities in access to care, but one that has been little studied. By definition, public health plays an important role in resolving disparities in health outcomes, access, and quality by performing three critical functions: assurance, assessment, and policymaking.

Public health can most directly influence health care disparities by assurance or oversight. In this role, public health links populations to needed health care services, ensures that a competent and diverse workforce exists, and evaluates the effectiveness, accessibility, and quality of the services delivered. In most cases, this involves providing immunizations, testing, and treatment for certain communicable diseases, identifying gaps in services, and providing community outreach. Assessment (or what is commonly termed surveillance activities) focuses on identifying specific health issues among particular segments of the population, such as colorectal cancer screening in adults 50–75 years of age, obesity among non-Hispanic Blacks, and blood pressure control among Mexican Americans. Once these health disparities are identified, local public health officials can work with providers and key stakeholders to address them in the communities where the problems reside. Finally, public health plays a leading role in developing policies covering everything from antismoking campaigns to promoting physical activity and the removal of lead from the environment.

Effectively addressing disparities in health and health care requires a collective effort that includes a partnership between public health, the health care system, and local community-based organizations (CBOs). Public health can also play an important convener role with other organizations and sectors, such as business, academe, and the media, by providing policy and administrative leaderships to strengthen such partnerships.

Policymakers

The elimination of health care disparities is politically sensitive and challenging in part because the causes of these disparities are intertwined with a contentious history of race relations in America. Nonetheless, the assurance of health equity is critically important to stakeholders, including health plans, payers, providers, and individuals. The US Congress provided early support by legislatively mandating the NAM study on health care disparities, creating the National Center on Minority Health and Health Disparities at the NIH, and requiring HHS to produce the *National Health Care Disparities Report* [8]. However, while attention to racial and ethnic disparities in care has increased among policymakers, there has been little consensus over the past decade on what can or should be done to reduce these gaps.

To date, most policymaking has centered on four broad areas: (1) raising public and provider awareness of racial/ethnic disparities in care; (2) expanding health insurance coverage; (3) increasing the number and type of providers in underserved communities; and (4) increasing the knowledge base on causes and interventions to reduce disparities. Results have been mixed across the four areas, with some success reported in increasing provider awareness and insurance coverage through the ACA Medicaid expansion. In its five-year strategic plan [23], HHS has identified three specific goals: (1) achieve health equity; (2) ensure access to quality, culturally competent care for vulnerable populations; and (3) improve data collection and measurement. While some progress has been made on the first two goals, much more advancement has been made on collecting, analyzing, and using new types of data to understand and address health and health care disparities. Under the Obama Administration, HHS released new, refined standards for capturing race, ethnicity, sex, primary language, and disability data. Work by the National Quality Foundation (NQF) has led to new consensus metrics becoming available to address health care disparities and cultural competency [24], while HHS continues to work with major stakeholders on developing policy and practice standards strengthening CLAS.

Hospitals, physicians, and health plans are now focused on capturing data to assess health care disparities. Three barriers encountered in this effort have policy ramifications. First, while most organizations say they are committed to this pursuit, making the business case to collect this data as part of normal operations is a much more difficult sell. Second, inconsistencies in the data and a lack of uniformity in the measures and tools limit the usability and quality of the data collected. Finally, data to define disparities among some subgroups—Native Americans (i.e., American Indians and Alaskan Natives) LGBT (Lesbian, Gay, Bisexual, and Transgender), military veterans, those living in rural areas and impoverished rural areas (e.g., Appalachia) and those with disabilities—are much more limited, if it exists at all [25].

The Dallas Experience

Over the past decade, Parkland Health and Hospital System (Parkland) and (more recently) the Parkland Center for Clinical Innovation (PCCI), have been developing a variety of community-facing programs, resources, and data tools to better understand the nature and scope of Dallas-area vulnerable, underserved populations and then to improve their health and reduce the health care disparities gap through work with local Community-Based (Social Service) Organizations (a.k.a, CBOs). Parkland and PCCI have worked closely with many CBOs providing food, housing, transportation, and crisis counseling services in some of the most impoverished areas of the city in order to understand both the clinical and social needs of the residents. Using a PCCI-developed readiness assessment tool and community data resource application, the CBOs were able to identify and quantify community needs down to the block level and then begin to match those needs with available community services. Central to the work of Parkland and PCCI has been the unwavering commitment to reduce the impact that SDOH have on vulnerable, underserved populations. Key to this effort was the development of the Dallas Information Exchange Portal (IEP), a pioneering electronic referral /case management platform funded through a grant from The W.W. Caruth, Jr. Foundation at Communities Foundation of Texas.

Created in 2014 by PCCI as a partnership between Parkland and a number of CBOs, the IEP was among the first cloud-based, case-management software applications to be built at scale to connect CBOs (and the vulnerable community residents they serve) with health care providers in a seamless and efficient manner. The IEP not only serves as a referral mechanism, allowing providers to send patients presenting in the ER with both medical issues and social needs (e.g., in need of food and/or shelter) to CBOs (e.g., local food pantries and/or homeless shelters), it allows the collection of vast amounts of non-PHI demographic and health data on the individuals making up these populations. With the patient's and network participant's consent, this information is made available to all entities that the individual comes in contact within the network to better understand and manage the patient's care. Over several years, PCCI has been able to identify and quantify profiles of the

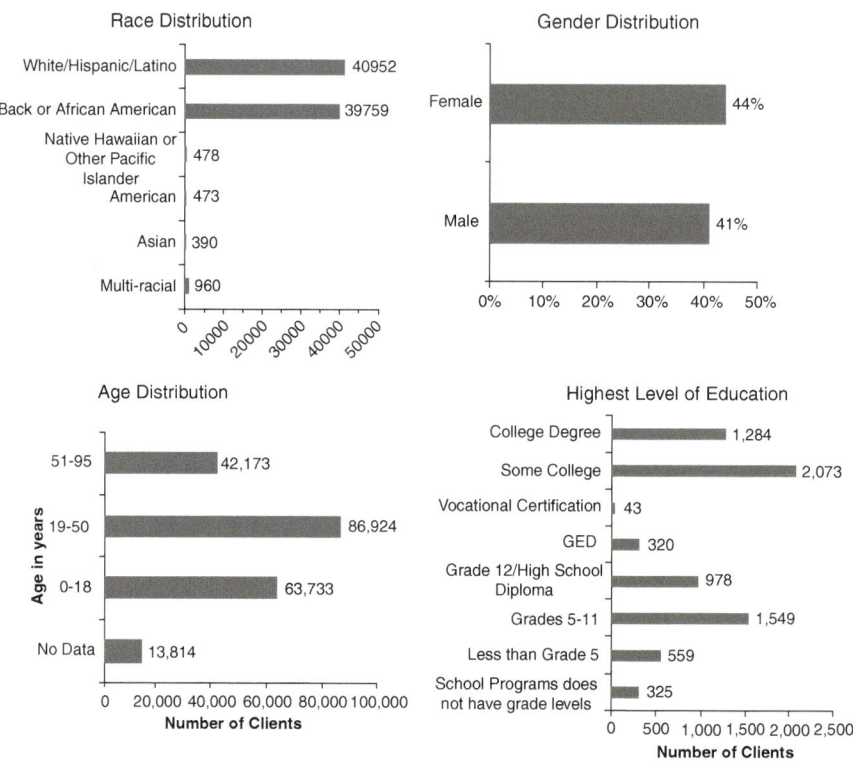

Fig. 7.1 Dallas IEP User Demographics, 2017

individuals using the IEP. Figure 7.1 presents a summary of some of the over one-hundred data elements (in this case, user demographics), collected by the Dallas IEP.

While the Dallas IEP has represented a quantum leap forward in understanding the makeup of vulnerable populations and providing an infrastructure for two-way communication between providers and CBOs, it wasn't until several years later that PCCI was able to fully document the nature and scope of SDOH needs among this population and the role these health-related social determinants play in fostering health and health care disparities. In 2017, the Center for Medicare and Medicaid Innovation (CMMI) within the US Department of Health and Human Services launched the Accountable Health Communities Model demonstration program [26] to determine if helping Medicare and Medicaid beneficiaries identify and address key upstream factors (i.e., health-related social determinants) would reduce inappropriate utilization of Emergency Departments and health care expenses. Central to this effort was the development by CMMI of a simple SDOH assessment screening tool that all demonstration sites (bridge organizations) were required to use to collect information on health-related social needs. Being one of thirty nationwide demonstration sites, PCCI incorporated the needs assessment screening tool into the IEP to link patients' clinical needs with their social needs. Data collected by PCCI in Dallas indicated that food was the highest reported need at 45%, followed by housing at 25%, transportation at 14%, utilities at 13%, and personal safety at 3% [27].[1]

While the recognition of SDOH needs and how these perpetuate disparities in health and health care is critically important, having the local resources and services available to meet those needs is equally important. The ongoing work done in Dallas and by other organizations in other communities across the country has documented the misalignment of social needs and available resources. It is not surprising that areas with the highest degree of SDOH needs are typically those with the fewest available resources because of their challenged urban or rural locations, historically identified by zip codes. More recent work by researchers has shown that zip codes are often not a reliable indicator as pronounced socioeconomic differences can exist within a given zip code. Understanding the need to quantify these misalignments as precisely as possible, PCCI developed an application that combines publicly available data with patient-level SDOH needs-assessment data to construct SDOH geo-map needs at the block level. These geo-maps can identify differences within a zip code at the block group level, providing a more granular picture of the community. For example, zip code 75202, commonly recognized as one of the most affluent areas in Dallas based on median household income, has several block groups (i.e., neighborhoods) within the zip code where median household income is near the federal poverty level for a family of four. These block group geo-maps are then linked with known CBOs and other local social service resources to create hot-spot maps for individual communities and neighborhoods within those communities.

The work of PCCI and its partners in Dallas is an example of how technology and a data-driven approach can be leveraged to better understand the upstream drivers of health and health care disparities among a large, vulnerable, and underserved urban population. The collection and use of REAL (race, ethnicity, and language) data are key requirements of the process of identifying and eliminating disparities. To be successful, we must ensure our data systems capture the appropriate categories of data consistently across different venues. More sophisticated data analytic tools and methods, along with greater standardization, are needed to support a burgeoning field of research on health inequities. Understanding, at the individual level, the economic, social, and environmental risk factors that give rise to, or perpetuate, the gaps seen between various groups within the population can be enhanced through the use of artificial intelligence and machine learning strategies that are now just being introduced to the discipline. Better, more representative data and advanced analytic techniques for evaluating that data will provide a strong foundation upon which to establish more effective policies and interventions to address health and health care disparities.

---

[1] The project described was supported by Funding Opportunity Number CMS-1P1-17-001 from the U.S. Department of Health & Human Services, Centers for Medicare & Medicaid Services. The contents provided are solely the responsibility of PCCI and do not necessarily represent the official views of HHS or any of its agencies.

While data will continue to play a key role in helping us understand and quantify the nature and scope of health and health care disparities, policymakers will also need to design innovative payment mechanisms to incent behaviors that reduce or eliminate disparities, while penalizing counterproductive actions. To be successful, these payment policies must be broad-based, touching all components of the continuum of care, including all those involved in delivering that care. These payment policies compound the disparity effect in the health care system in which certain entities, such as safety net hospitals, typically care for some of the most vulnerable individuals. Adjustments must be made to current rules, such as penalties for readmission rates and 30-day mortality rates for this unique population mix, to keep from unfairly penalizing providers treating a disproportionate share of vulnerable and underserved populations.

Finally, the experience in Dallas has shown the need for collaboration and meaningful partnerships between health care providers and social service organizations along with researchers and health system innovation stakeholders. The health care system alone cannot solve the problem of health and health care disparities, although they play a large contributory role. Similarly, social service organizations cannot single-handedly solve the problem because of their limited financial resources. With the help of local/state public health agencies and policymaking at the state and national levels, health and health care disparities could be virtually eliminated if the issue is viewed as a national priority. Anything short of that will likely result in continued gaps in care and health status for a large segment of our population.

Conclusions

Despite some substantial strides, significant and unacceptable health and health care disparities continue to persist in the United States, leading to certain groups at higher risk of being uninsured, having limited access to care, and experiencing poorer outcomes. While health and health care disparities are frequently seen in terms of race and ethnicity, they occur across a broad range of dimensions and reflect a complex set of social, environmental, and individual factors. Moreover, they not only impact those facing an uneven playing field but limit the health and economic prosperity of the entire society. As the racial, ethnic, and demographic composition of society changes, it becomes increasingly important to understand and reduce the gaps between population groups.

Since the release of the Heckler Report [5], the United States has increased its focus on reducing disparities, with a growing set of policies, initiatives, and government agencies created to bring about positive change. While many of these efforts have shown promise and progress, much work remains. Direct or implicit bias persists within many provider encounters, while the number of minority providers, faculty, and researchers remains woefully low. Our understanding of many US subgroups and group-specific diseases remains rudimentary due to a lack of meaningful data. In addition, an overall awareness of health and health care disparities remains surprisingly low among the general public.

Several goal-directed, future initiatives hold great promise in reducing health and health care disparities. These include:

- Building infrastructure, including sustainability funding to support local interventions
- Aligning policy and payment mechanisms with goals of reducing disparities
- Expansion of efforts, including health disparity measures and indices, to cover other groups, such as Native Americans, Asian-Pacific Islanders, LGBT, people with disabilities, and military veterans
- Expansion of metrics to capture the broader definition of health, including health equity and the SDOH
- Establishment of longer-term studies to document quantifiable changes in health outcomes related to disparities and SDOH.

Even with these progressive initiatives, the future health of the US populace will be determined to a large extent by how effectively federal, state, and local agencies and private organizations work with communities to reduce or eliminate health and health care disparities among those populations experiencing a disproportionate burden of disease, disability, and death.

References/Associated Reading

1. National Institutes of Health. Health disparities, 2014. http://www.nhlbi.nih.gov/health/educational/healthdisp.
2. Graham H. Social determinants and their unequal distribution: clarifying policy understandings. Milbank Q. 2004;82(1):101–24.
3. Woolf SH, Aron L. U.S. Health in international perspective: shorter lives, poorer health. Washington, DC: The National Academies Press; 2013.
4. Grant JM, Mottet LA, Tanis J. National transgender discrimination survey: report on health and health care. Washington, DC: National Center for Transgender Equality and the National Gay and Lesbian Task Force; 2010.
5. Heckler MM, Report of the secretary's task force on black and minority health, United States Department of Health and Human Services, 1985.
6. Smedley BD, Stith AY, Nelson AR. Unequal treatment: confronting racial and ethnic disparities in health care. Washington, DC: The National Academies Press; 2003.
7. Centers for Disease Control and Prevention. Surveillance of health status in minority communities- Racial and Ethnic Approaches to Community Health across the U.S. (REACH U.S.) risk factor survey, 2009.
8. U.S. Department of Health & Human Services. National healthcare disparities report, Department of Health & Human Services, Washington, DC, 2012.
9. Joint Center for Political and Economic Studies. The economic burden of health inequities in the United States, Washington, DC, 2009.
10. Turner A. The business case for racial equity, a strategy for growth: WK Kellogg Foundation and Altarum; 2018. http://altarum.org/publications//the-business-case-for-racial-equity-a-strategy-for-growth.
11. Centers for Disease Control and Prevention. Health disparities and inequalities report-United States, 2013. MMWR. 2013;62(suppl.3):1–187.
12. National Center for Health Statistics. Healthy people two thousand ten final review. Hyattsville: National Center for Health Statistics; 2012.

13. Agency for Healthcare Research and Quality. 2016 National healthcare quality and disparities report, agency for healthcare research and quality, Rockville, 2017.
14. Orgera K, Artiga S. Disparities in health and health care: five key questions and answers. San Francisco: Henry J. Kaiser Family Foundation; 2018.
15. Riley WJ. Health disparities: gaps in access, quality, and affordability of medical care. Trans Am Clin Climatol Assoc. 2012;123:167–74.
16. Budhwani H, Hearld K, Chavez-Yenter D. Depression in racial and ethnic minorities: the impact of nativity and discrimination. Racial Ethn Health Disparities. 2015;2(1):34–42.
17. Henry J. Kaiser Family Foundation and the American College of Cardiology. Report on racial/ethnic differences in cardiac care: the weight of the evidence, San Francisco, 2002.
18. Whittle J, Conigliaro J, Good CB, Lofgren RP. Racial differences in the use of invasive cardiovascular procedures in the Department of Veterans Affairs Medical System. N Engl J Med. 1993;329:621–7.
19. U.S. Department of Health & Human Services. HHS action plan to reduce racial and ethnic health disparities: a nation free of disparities in health and health care. Washington, DC: Department of Health & Human Services; 2011. www.hhs.gov/strategic-plan/eliminate.html.
20. Hayes SL, Riley P, Radley DC, McCarthy D. Reducing racial and ethnic disparities in access to care: has the Affordable Care Act made a difference? Commonwealth Fund Issues Briefs, 2017, Aug 1–16.
21. Hall WJ, Chapman MV, Lee KM, et al. Implicit racial/ethnic bias among health care professionals and its influence on health care outcomes. Am J Public Health. 2015;105(12):e60–76.
22. Phillips JM, Malone B. Increasing racial/ethnic diversity in nursing to reduce health disparities and achieve health equity. Public Health Rep. 2014;129(Suppl 2):45–50.
23. U.S. Department of Health & Human Services Strategic Plan 2010-2015, Department of Health & Human Services, Washington DC, 2010.
24. National Quality Forum. Endorsement summary: healthcare disparities and cultural competency measures. Washington, DC: National Quality Forum; 2012, Aug.
25. Baciu A, Negussie Y, Geller A, et al. The State of health disparities in the United States. Washington, DC: National Academies Press; 2017.
26. Center for Medicare and Medicaid Innovation. Accountable health communities model. www.innovation.cms.gov.
27. PCCI's March 1, 2019 Progress report submitted to W.W. Caruth, Jr. Foundation fund at Communities Foundation of Texas, covering program activities between 3/1/2018 through 2/28/2019.

Preventing Mistakes in Health Care

8

Pranavi V. Sreeramoju

The basic tenet of medicine is "first, do no harm." Almost no one in health care goes to work thinking that s/he will harm a patient who is in his or her care on any given day. Yet, per the Harvard Medical Practice Study published in 1991, an estimated 3.7% of hospital patients have disabling injuries caused by medical treatment. As noted in the chapter on current landscape of quality, publications by the National Academies highlighting medical errors [1] and the "quality chasm" [2] got the attention of health care professional community as well as the public. Estimates of the number of people who die annually in the US from medical errors range from 44,000–98,000 deaths per the National Academies publications to over 400,000 deaths per year per a study using a different methodology [3]. The absence of harm in health care is called patient safety. The types of health care safety events that we recognize and strive to prevent have evolved substantially over the last few decades. While medication errors [4], health care-associated infections [5], and surgical complications were among the earliest errors recognized in health care, events such as venous thromboembolism, falls, pressure ulcers and, most recently, diagnostic errors [6, 7] have gained attention. In this chapter, the terms mistakes, errors, safety events, adverse events, and patient harm are used interchangeably, although there are some important differences. While both mistakes and errors are a result of wrong action proceeding from faulty judgment, inadequate knowledge, or inattention, for a mistake, there is usually, recognition that what occurred is incorrect whereas for an error, such recognition may not be present. This chapter is intended to be an overview of how patient safety is approached in hospitals and health care systems and a call to action for patients, professionals in health care, policymakers, payers, and the public. Strategies to prevent individual types of safety events are not discussed. Health care personnel safety events such as needlestick injuries are beyond the scope of this chapter.

P. V. Sreeramoju (✉)
Department of Internal Medicine, UT Southwestern Medical Center, Dallas, TX, USA
e-mail: Pranavi.Sreeramoju@UTSouthwestern.edu

© Springer Nature Switzerland AG 2020
P. V. Sreeramoju et al. (eds.), *The Patient and Health Care System: Perspectives on High-Quality Care*, https://doi.org/10.1007/978-3-030-46567-4_8

A major reason for safety events in modern medicine is the increasing complexity of care provided in the twenty-first century [8] and the increasing number of people involved in caring for each patient, which is particularly true for patients in intensive care units and those undergoing surgery [9, 10]. As noted previously by several patient safety experts, some of the safety issues may be a "problem of many hands." Inability to hold an individual or a team accountable for safety outcomes can be problematic. A typical "inter-professional," "multi-disciplinary" patient care team has several members each with a "deep area of specialization" who may or may not have the skills to communicate and coordinate with other members of the team. Care protocols unique to individual specialties (e.g., cardiology, infectious diseases, plastic surgery) and professionals (e.g., physicians, nurses, respiratory therapists) may not seamlessly flow into each other when they receive care from the patient care team as a whole. Donald Berwick, in his thoughtful paper on controlling variation in health care, discusses the "illusion of control" [11]. He writes: "They (health care personnel) are not, however, in control of their work. Like me, they push at the sides of the work, nudging it toward the perfection they really desire, and, like me, they feel it move only ever so slightly in response to their strenuous efforts. They want it to be better; but they do not know how to make it so."

Mistakes in health care have a sharp end and a latent or system end. While mistakes at the sharp end show as harm to the patient, mistakes at the latent end constitute the multitude of conditions in the health care system that allow mistakes to occur. A model that may help understand the conditions, which constitute the "system end," is the Swiss cheese model originally articulated by James Reason [12, 13]. In this model, organizational influences, such as culture and leadership, unsafe supervision, preconditions for lack of safety, and the unsafe acts themselves are like slices of Swiss cheese; when the "eyes" align, the mistake passes through the imperfect layers and reaches the patient. For example, when a health care-associated infection occurs in a patient, the sharp end of the mistake is the infection that occurred. At the system end, there could be lapses in hand hygiene, insufficiencies in use of sterile barrier precautions and central line kits, inadequate culture of safety and leadership, or very rarely, egregious and reckless violation of infection prevention protocols. Similarly, while a wrong site surgery is at the sharp end, lack of processes to mark site correctly, lack of proper hand off procedures between different teams, lack of accountability, personnel burnout and insufficient culture of safety and psychological safety for calling out mistakes could be at the latent end of the error. Monitoring these mistakes in health care systems requires standardized surveillance.

Measurement of Safety in Health Care

Measurement and data are foundational to improving patient safety in health care. In patient safety history, Ignaz Semmelweis [14], Florence Nightingale [15], and Ernest Codman [16] demonstrated using data that patient safety outcomes improved with the implementation of specific interventions. In modern health care, patient safety is measured with the use of several metrics. Some examples are below.

- Outcome measures: Patient safety indicators such as pressure ulcer, iatrogenic pneumothorax, postoperative sepsis; Total hip and knee arthroplasty associated complications; Rates of health care-associated infections such as central line-associated blood stream infection, catheter-associated urinary tract infection, surgical site infection after colon surgery or hysterectomy, methicillin-resistant *Staphylococcus aureus*, *Clostridioides difficile* infection; Incidence of medication errors; Rate of falls
- Process measures: Hand hygiene adherence; Medication reconciliation; Antimicrobial usage
- Satisfaction measures: Satisfaction with cleanliness of environment; Satisfaction with discharge instructions
- Surrogate measures: Hospital culture of safety survey; Safety attitudes questionnaire

With increasing discovery in the area of patient safety, the number and type of metrics used by several organizations has increased organically. The National Academies in their report, "Vital signs: Core metrics for health and health care progress," [17] describe the unsustainability of the large number of measurements that currently exist. Per the report, patient safety is measured with the use of 97 metrics, with 42 being publically reported. Organizations to whom safety data are reported include the Centers for Medicare and Medicaid Services (CMS), The Joint Commission (TJC), Leapfrog, National Committee for Quality Assurance, and the Office of the National Coordinator for Health Information Technology. The report emphasizes the need for leadership at every level to make patient safety measurement more efficient.

Within each health care system, the best practice is to use an event reporting system that allows organizational learning and allows leadership to address patient safety systematically. Everyone working in the organization, including the physicians, nurses, trainees, and other professionals are strongly encouraged to report every safety event that they have encountered in their routine practice. The report is assumed to be made in good faith. The American Society of Health Care Risk and Management recommends using the following scale [18] for harm events occurring in health care facilities.

- A—Death: Dead at time of assessment
- B—Severe harm: Bodily or psychological injury (including pain or disfigurement) that interferes significantly with functional ability or quality of life
- C—Moderate harm: Bodily or psychological injury adversely affecting functional ability or quality of life, but not at the level of severe harm
- D—Mild harm: Minimal symptoms or loss of function, or injury limited to additional treatment, monitoring, and/or increased length of stay
- E—No harm: Event reached patient, but no harm was evident

- F—Unknown

Data show that while progress with patient safety in US health care facilities is slower than expected, there is progress [19], particularly in the area of health care-associated infections [20] and medication safety [21]. Improvements have been a result of ongoing discovery and implementation of person-level and organization-level strategies.

Person-Level Strategies to Improve Patient Safety

Teamwork and Communication Strategies: The vast majority of person-level strategies to improve patient safety include training on teamwork and communication strategies. Notable teamwork training courses include Crew Resource Management [22] and TeamSTEPPS® [23]. Health care personnel are trained on team skills such as briefs, huddles, debriefs, coordination, and delegation. They are frequently trained in communication strategies such as

- Two Challenge rule (invoked when an initial assertion is ignored after voicing a concern assertively, and if the outcome is not acceptable, taking a stronger course of action such as stop the line)
- See it – Say it – Fix it, also called the "Southwest Airlines" way of calling attention to safety issues
- SBAR: Situation- Background- Assessment- Recommendations
- DESC Script for managing and resolving conflict: Describe the specific situation, Express your concerns about the action, Suggest other alternatives, and Consequences should be stated
- CUS: "I am Concerned" – "I am Uncomfortable" – "This is a Safety issue"

These communication tools improve effectiveness of communication and calling attention to safety issues in a constructive manner, in addition to improving psychological safety for speaking up. Health care systems, particularly academic medical centers, tend to be hierarchical in nature. In addition, physicians depend on each other for referrals, and junior physicians and trainees depend on other physicians for opportunities, which creates conditions for lack of psychological safety to speak up. Rana Awdish [24], in a particularly emotional and insightful account of the safety events that happened to her when she was hospitalized as a patient where she was a physician trainee, she describes a resident who ordered an incorrect medication in spite of his better judgment because he did not want to speak up to the attending physician. Even when psychological safety exists, health care personnel must navigate differences in race, color, social and cultural backgrounds, language proficiency, and linguistic styles, in order to communicate with each other effectively. Safety events are personal to the patient as well as to the health care teams, and organizations that implemented programs to provide support and counseling to the health care personnel involved in the safety event, called "second victims," [25] are promising to improve physician burnout and patient care. While strategies to improve personal effectiveness and team effectiveness in health care are relatively well developed, strategies to address teamwork and coordination among "teams of teams" are relatively less developed. A particularly promising approach is relational coordination [26], which is based on findings that seven aspects of a relationship between teams, i.e., timeliness, accuracy, frequency, and problem-solving nature of communication; and shared respect, shared goals, and shared knowledge, have a positive impact on outcomes. Multiple teams working in parallel care for most patients. Therefore, it is extremely critical for health care systems to address teamwork between teams.

Critical Thinking: Preventability of safety events largely depends on risk anticipation, and clinicians are constantly weighing risks and benefits for every decision made in patient care. The need to teach critical thinking and train in reduction of cognitive biases is being recognized in health care with the goal of reducing diagnostic errors and incorrect management decisions [27]. Physicians as well as patients need to recognize and embrace uncertainty in clinical medicine, rather than think that it is a sign of ignorance or incompetence.

Leadership and Followership: Much attention is being given to leadership in health care and, consequently, investments in leadership training are integral to improving patient safety. At a person-level, leadership in clinical medicine independent of having a designated leadership role is key, particularly in complex or tension-filled situations [28]. On the other hand, followership is less understood in health care. Leung and others write in their review article [29] on the topic, "Followership can be difficult to define, but generally depends upon the processes by which people follow, who they follow, and how much engagement and influence they exert." Per Kelley, there are five types of followership styles: passive, conformist, alienated, pragmatists, and effective followers [30]. It remains to be understood how leadership styles and followership styles correlate with medical errors, infection rates, satisfaction, and team resilience.

Mastery: Lastly, person-level approaches to improve patient safety must focus on mastery of skills, along with meaning that motivated clinicians to embark on a journey in medicine in the first place. Approaches to improve mindfulness [31], meaning [32], and mastery might reduce burnout and cause greater physician satisfaction. In his essay "Personal Best," [33] Atul Gawande makes a strong case for physicians and surgeons to have coaches, similar to top athletes and singers, because mastery is about familiarity and judgment. Learning to head off problems individually and in teams is the best way to provide clinical care in a safe manner.

Organization-Level Approaches to Improve Patient Safety

The science of safety evolved from the days of implementing hand washing in the postpartum ward during the days of Semmelweis at the expense of anger and ridicule from the medical establishment of the day to the use of checklists [34–36] and sophisticated sociotechnical approaches [37, 38] and continues to evolve. Some key concepts below describe how safety is addressed in health care systems today.

Culture: An organization's culture is based on shared attitudes, beliefs, customs, and written and unwritten rules that have been developed over time. In a patient safety culture model [39], organizational culture reflects core values that inform patient safety culture, which in turn create a patient safety climate that drives an individual's attitudes and behaviors towards patient safety. Per the Agency for Health Care Research and Quality, an organization's commitment to patient safety is reflected in these key actions: acknowledgment of the high-risk nature of an organization's activities and the determination to achieve consistently safe operations, a blame-free environment where individuals are able to report errors or near misses without fear of reprimand or punishment, encouragement of collaboration across ranks and disciplines to seek solutions to patient safety problems, and organizational commitment of resources to address safety concerns [40]. In modern times, it is widely acknowledged that intentional effort to improve culture of safety is necessary to make an organization safer [41]. Creating psychological safety is necessary for health care personnel to speak up against unsafe practices. Interventions that show promise in improving culture of safety include team training, unit-based safety teams, positive deviance to identify barriers and seek solutions from the bedside, and executive walk rounds to engage staff and patients in daily goal setting [41, 42].

Just Culture: To evaluate personal failures and behavior choices of health care personnel who fail to use safe patient care practices (e.g., hand hygiene), a just culture framework [43] is used. Per just culture, negative behaviors in health care manifest across a spectrum: inadvertent action, or human error, behavior that is mistakenly believed to be justified, also known as at-risk behavior, and behavior choice that consciously ignores a substantial risk, otherwise known as reckless behavior. Classifying unsafe behaviors in this manner provides a framework for judging each behavior and determine an appropriate response. Consoling the staff member may be adequate for inadvertent actions; coaching is needed for at-risk behaviors, and punishment may be necessary for reckless behavior. These principles help organizations deal with difficult situations in which the generally appropriate focus on systems needs to be shifted towards individual accountability.

High reliability: To achieve consistency of practice, organizations need to embrace principles of high reliability organizations [44]. The five principles of high-reliability organizations are preoccupation with failure, embracing complexity and reluctance to simplify, commitment to resilience, sensitivity to operations, and deference to expertise. To be called highly reliable, an organization must demonstrate leadership, robust process improvement, and a safety culture. Examples of national programs that reward high reliability are Get With The Guidelines® [45] by the American Heart Association for stroke, heart failure, coronary artery disease, atrial fibrillation, and resuscitation. As one might expect, execution is key at all levels to achieve high reliability of practice.

Root cause analysis: In order to evaluate errors that occurred, root cause analyses (RCA) are conducted to identify fundamental problems and vulnerabilities in the system and implement preventive measures to prevent future harm [46]. The National Patient Safety Foundation developed a more advanced approach to evaluating errors called the RCA^2 [47]. The method uses improvement science to implement engineering controls, standardization, and uses a hierarchy of actions that allows prioritization of stronger actions (e.g., physical plant changes) over weaker actions (e.g., in-service training, policy memoranda).

Failure Mode and Effects Analysis: Another approach in patient safety to anticipate and analyze all possible modes of failure in order to identify and implement measures to prevent failure is called Failure Mode and Effects Analysis (FMEA) [48]. For example, an FMEA may be conducted when opening an influenza unit in the emergency department during peak flu season to handle the surge in cases.

Human Factors Analysis and Classification System: The approach facilitates systematic evaluation of errors involving humans and focuses on why an error may have occurred [49]. Human factors leading up to an error—organizational influences, supervisory factors, preconditions for unsafe acts including conditions of operators (mental states, physiological states, and physical/mental limitations)—are analyzed. Errors are recognized as being due to coordination, communication, or skill-based error.

Work and Workplace Redesign: The architectural design of health care facilities, technology, including digital health technology, equipment, and functionality of the spaces have a substantial impact on patient safety and overall quality of care. A good design addresses human factors and prevents inadvertent errors [50, 51], also called mistake proofing or poka-yoke (e.g., having separate and differently marked windows for delivery of dirty instruments and picking up clean instruments in the sterile processing department).

Patient Advocacy, Media, and Patient Safety

Patient and caregiver advocacy and the media have shaped the patient safety movement in several ways over the years. Sorrel King, a mom who turned into a strong advocate for patient safety, tells a particularly impactful story [52]. Her eighteen-month-old daughter, Josie King, was burned by hot water in a bathtub due to a faulty water heater at home, and admitted to the hospital for care. This was back in 2001. She healed from the burn injuries and just before she was set to be discharged home, she developed a central line-associated bloodstream infection. Several "mistakes" happened in rather quick succession. The resulting sepsis caused decreased renal function, which required her pain medication to be adjusted for the newly decreased function. However, she received a dose that is correct for patients with normal renal function, and she developed symptoms of pain medication overdose, which required "reversal" with a different medication called naloxone. Later, during the child's hospital stay, in spite of a "verbal order" to not give her any more narcotic pain medications, a nurse gave her narcotic, which resulted in a code and subsequent death. Because of Sorrel King's advocacy, the medical center where these harm events occurred now has a robust patient safety program and the leadership lessons learned from her devastating experience were impactful throughout the patient safety community in the world.

In contrast to Sorrel King, Dennis Quaid was a celebrity when his ten-day old twins were harmed during their hospital stay because of a medical mistake [53]. The twins were given a dose of heparin that was 1000 times the correct dose because the packaging of the two doses of heparin was not different enough. These "Sound-Alike Look-Alike Drugs," or SALAD drugs as they are referred to, have contributed to numerous medication administration mistakes in health care. The actor went on to successfully sue the drug manufacturer and make a series of documentaries on patient safety. Luckily for him, his twins survived the medical mistake and they are teenagers as of this writing, unlike several other children who did not survive a similar mistake.

In a very insightful article, "Pushing the profession: how the news media turned patient safety into a priority," [54] Millenson discusses diffusion of innovation in medical error reduction and the role of outside pressure in changing ingrained thinking. In addition to bringing news to the public, they create awareness, amplify public health and patient safety messages, and foster meaningful advocacy and activism. Media stories that seek sensationalism and those with accusatory overtones are not helpful. Holding health care systems and clinicians accountable for medical mistakes and errors should not come at the cost of undermining confidence in them.

Public Programs in Place to Incentivize Safety in Health Care

There are several federal and state programs in place to ensure safety of patient care in hospitals. Hospital licensing and accreditation is contingent on meeting The Joint Commission national patient safety goals and the conditions of participation of the Centers for Medicare and Medicaid Services. The Accreditation Council for Graduate Medical Education has a program called Clinical Learning Environment Review that provides feedback to residency programs on patient safety, in addition to quality, care transitions, supervision, well-being, and professionalism. Public reporting of hospital data allows for greater transparency. Leapfrog gives a safety grade to hospitals based on their performance. The Centers for Medicare and Medicaid Services's value-based programs incentivize improvements in patient safety.

Closing Thoughts and a Call to Action

Humans are inherently error-prone, but with sufficient awareness, engagement, training, and reinforcement of safety behaviors and practices, health systems can become even safer than they currently are. Clinical outcomes and processes that were previously considered inevitable are now considered preventable errors and mistakes. New frontiers, such as safety in outpatient areas and digital health technologies, are being explored. The science of patient safety continues to evolve and it takes all parties to be continually open-minded. Even though "the system" may seem too complex and daunting, leaving little room for individual accountability, the system is made of individuals. Patient safety in a health care system is a function of each individual doing what is safe for the patient in a coordinated manner. Below are some suggested actions for each of the stakeholders.

Patients
- Become familiar with your rights as a patient.
- Be aware of the care you are getting, e.g., visits, labs, medications. If something doesn't seem right, (e.g., a clinician not performing hand hygiene) feel free to speak up or go to patient relations or consider getting yourself a patient advocate. Speak up if something doesn't seem right.
- Review whether the health care experience is meeting your needs and, if not, consider calling attention to your needs. Members of the health care team may have different ideas and values compared to you; know that it is within your rights that they hear what is important to you.
- Feel free to ask questions and, to the extent possible, be an active participant in your care. Resources for how patients and caregivers can help prevent medication-related and other errors are available from organizations like The Joint Commission and the Agency for Health Care Research in Quality [55, 56].

Clinicians
- Stay educated about safety protocols and use them routinely in clinical care.
- Apply critical thinking and mindfulness—rare patient safety events do not always have a protocol for prevention.
- Know who your partners in patient safety are.
- Learn and use team training and communication skills; practice situational leadership.
- Model safety behaviors and encourage peers to do the same. Positive peer pressure is a healthy force in advancing patient safety.
- Report errors, participate in root cause analyses and action planning as needed.
- Step forward to leadership roles in patient safety when needs arise.
- Patients and families are part of your safety team; Seek their input actively regarding any incident that "does not seem right."

Administrators
- Invest in a robust patient safety program for the organization.
- Implement programs to improve patient safety culture in the organization.
- Invest resources in information systems and automating workflows that enable "mistake-proofing."
- Monitor for and prevent "siloing" between systems, departments, and services.
- Participate in patient safety collaboratives.
- Invest in training and research on patient safety.

Payors

- Provide incentives for good performance on patient safety.
- Generate meaningful data and share data with providers.

Policymakers

- Align incentives and disincentives well.
- Pass laws that allow for sound investments in infrastructures and research. Research in patient safety is underfunded and undersupported. For example, NIH annual budget was around $30 billion and AHRQ annual budget was around $400 million in 2018.

References

1. Kohn LT, Corrigan J, Donaldson MS. To err is human: building a safer health system. Washington, D.C.: National Academy Press; 2000.
2. Crossing the quality chasm: a new health system for the 21st century. Washington, DC: The National Academies Press; 2001. https://doi.org/10.17226/10027.
3. Makary MA, Daniel M. Medical error-the third leading cause of death in the US. BMJ. 2016;353:i2139.
4. Keers RN, Williams SD, Cooke J, Ashcroft DM. Causes of medication administration errors in hospitals: a systematic review of quantitative and qualitative evidence. Drug Saf. 2013;36(11):1045–67.
5. The Centers for Disease Control and Prevention; Available from: https://www.cdc.gov/hai/index.html.
6. Newman-Toker DE, Pronovost PJ. Diagnostic errors--the next frontier for patient safety. JAMA. 2009;301(10):1060–2.
7. Singh H, Meyer AN, Thomas EJ. The frequency of diagnostic errors in outpatient care: estimations from three large observational studies involving US adult populations. BMJ Qual Saf. 2014;23(9):727–31.
8. Jha A. The real cause of deadly medical errors 2016. Available from: https://blogs.scientificamerican.com/guest-blog/the-real-cause-of-deadly-medical-errors/.
9. Lark ME, Kirkpatrick K, Chung KC. Patient safety movement: history and future directions. J Hand Surg Am. 2018;43(2):174–8.
10. Makary MA, Sexton JB, Freischlag JA, Millman EA, Pryor D, Holzmueller C, et al. Patient safety in surgery. Ann Surg. 2006;243(5):628–32; discussion 32-5.
11. Berwick DM. Controlling variation in health care: a consultation from Walter Shewhart. Med Care. 1991;29(12):1212–25.
12. Reason J. Understanding adverse events: human factors. Qual health care. 1995;4(2):80–9.
13. Reason J. Human error: models and management. West J Med. 2000;172(6):393–6.
14. Kadar N. Rediscovering Ignaz Philipp Semmelweis (1818-1865). Am J Obstet Gynecol. 2019;220(1):26–39.
15. Aravind M, Chung KC. Evidence-based medicine and hospital reform: tracing origins back to Florence Nightingale. Plast Reconstr Surg. 2010;125(1):403–9.
16. Neuhauser D. Ernest Amory Codman MD. Qual Saf health care. 2002;11(1):104–5.
17. Blumenthal D, Malphrus E, McGinnis JM, editors. Vital signs: core metrics for health and health care progress. Washington, DC: The National Academies Press; 2015.
18. Hoppes M, Mitchell JL, Venditti EG, Bunting RF Jr. Serious safety events: getting to zero. J Healthc Risk Manag. 2013;32(3):27–45.

19. Pronovost PJ, Wachter RM. Progress in patient safety: a glass fuller than it seems. Am J Med Qual. 2014;29(2):165–9.
20. 2018 National and State Healthcare-Associated Infections Progress Report: Centers for Disease Control and Prevention; Available from: https://www.cdc.gov/hai/data/portal/progress-report.html.
21. Bates DW, Singh H. Two decades since to err is human: an assessment of progress and emerging priorities in patient safety. Health Aff (Millwood). 2018;37(11):1736–43.
22. Gross B, Rusin L, Kiesewetter J, Zottmann JM, Fischer MR, Pruckner S, et al. Crew resource management training in healthcare: a systematic review of intervention design, training conditions and evaluation. BMJ Open. 2019;9(2):e025247.
23. TeamSTEPPS 2.0.: Agency for Healthcare Research and Quality, Rockville; [updated June 2019. Available from: https://www.ahrq.gov/teamstepps/index.html.
24. Awdish R. In shock: my journey from death to recovery and the redemptive power of hope: St. New York: Martin's Press.
25. Ozeke O, Ozeke V, Coskun O, Budakoglu II. Second victims in health care: current perspectives. Adv Med Educ Pract. 2019;10:593–603.
26. Collaborative RCR. Available from: https://heller.brandeis.edu/relational-coordination/.
27. Royce CS, Hayes MM, Schwartzstein RM. Teaching critical thinking: a case for instruction in cognitive biases to reduce diagnostic errors and improve patient safety. Acad Med. 2019;94(2):187–94.
28. Roussel L. Leadership's impact on quality, outcomes, and costs. Crit Care Nurs Clin North Am. 2019;31(2):153–63.
29. Leung C, Lucas A, Brindley P, Anderson S, Park J, Vergis A, et al. Followership: a review of the literature in healthcare and beyond. J Crit Care. 2018;46:99–104.
30. Kelley RE. The power of followership : how to create leaders people want to follow, and followers who lead themselves. 1st ed; 1992.
31. Graling PR, Sanchez JA. Learning and mindfulness: improving perioperative patient safety. AORN J. 2017;105(3):317–21.
32. Hipp DM, Rialon KL, Nevel K, Kothari AN, Jardine LDA. "Back to bedside": residents' and fellows' perspectives on finding meaning in work. J Grad Med Educ. 2017;9(2):269–73.
33. Gawande A. Personal best: The New Yorker; 2011. Available from: https://www.newyorker.com/magazine/2011/10/03/personal-best.
34. Pronovost P, Needham D, Berenholtz S, Sinopoli D, Chu H, Cosgrove S, et al. An intervention to decrease catheter-related bloodstream infections in the ICU. N Engl J Med. 2006;355(26):2725–32.
35. Haynes AB, Weiser TG, Berry WR, Lipsitz SR, Breizat AH, Dellinger EP, et al. A surgical safety checklist to reduce morbidity and mortality in a global population. N Engl J Med. 2009;360(5):491–9.
36. Gawande A. The checklist manifesto: how to get things right. New York: Henry Holt and Company; 2009.
37. Sreeramoju P. Preventing healthcare-associated infections: beyond best practice. Am J Med Sci. 2013;345(3):239–44.
38. Sreeramoju P. Reducing infections "together": a review of socioadaptive approaches. Open Forum Infect Dis. 2019;6(2):ofy348.
39. Morello RT, Lowthian JA, Barker AL, McGinnes R, Dunt D, Brand C. Strategies for improving patient safety culture in hospitals: a systematic review. BMJ Qual Saf. 2013;22(1):11–8.
40. Culture of safety: Agency for Healthcare Research and Quality. Available from: https://psnet.ahrq.gov/primer/culture-safety.
41. Sreeramoju P, Dura L, Fernandez ME, Minhajuddin A, Simacek K, Fomby TB, et al. Using a positive deviance approach to influence the culture of patient safety related to infection prevention. Open Forum Infect Dis. 2018;5(10):ofy231.
42. Weaver SJ, Lubomksi LH, Wilson RF, Pfoh ER, Martinez KA, Dy SM. Promoting a culture of safety as a patient safety strategy: a systematic review. Ann Intern Med. 2013;158(5 Pt 2):369–74.

43. Marx D. Patient safety and the just culture: a primer for health care executives. New York: Trustees of Columbia University; 2001.
44. Chassin MR, Loeb JM. The ongoing quality improvement journey: next stop, high reliability. Health Aff (Millwood). 2011;30(4):559–68.
45. Association AH. Get with the Guidelines®. Available from: https://www.heart.org/en/professional/quality-improvement.
46. Charles R, Hood B, Derosier JM, Gosbee JW, Li Y, Caird MS, et al. How to perform a root cause analysis for workup and future prevention of medical errors: a review. Patient Saf Surg. 2016;10:20.
47. NPSF. NPSF. RCA2: improving root cause analyses and actions to prevent harm. Boston; 2015.
48. Ashley L, Armitage G, Neary M, Hollingsworth G. A practical guide to failure mode and effects analysis in health care: making the most of the team and its meetings. Jt Comm J Qual Patient Saf. 2010;36(8):351–8.
49. Diller T, Helmrich G, Dunning S, Cox S, Buchanan A, Shappell S. The Human Factors Analysis Classification System (HFACS) applied to health care. Am J Med Qual. 2014;29(3):181–90.
50. Reiling J, Hughes RG, Murphy MR. The impact of facility design on patient safety. In: Hughes RG, editor. Patient safety and quality: an evidence-based handbook for nurses. Advances in patient safety. Rockville; 2008.
51. Keeping patients safe: transforming the work environment of nurses. New York: National Academies Press; 2004.
52. King S. Josie's story: a Mother's inspiring crusade to make medical care safe. 1st ed. New York: Atlantic Monthly Press; 2009, Sept 8.
53. Arnquist S. Dennis Quaid takes on hospital errors 2008. Available from: https://thehealthcare-blog.com/blog/2008/03/28/dennis-quaid-takes-on-hospital-errors/.
54. Millenson ML. Pushing the profession: how the news media turned patient safety into a priority. Qual Saf health care. 2002;11(1):57–63.
55. 20 tips to help prevent medical errors: patient fact sheet: Agency for healthcare research and quality. Available from: https://www.ahrq.gov/patients-consumers/care-planning/errors/20tips/index.html.
56. Michael F. Roizen MO. YOU: the smart patient: an insider's handbook for getting the best treatment: Scribner; 2006.

Timeliness of Care

9

Stephen J. Harder and Eugene S. Chu

Introduction

Timeliness of care is defined by the National Academy of Medicine as "reducing waits and sometimes harmful delays for both those who receive and those who give care" [1]. Whether the lack of timeliness occurs in the evaluation or the treatment phase of health care, either can lead to adverse outcomes. Delays in care can further be contextualized into delays of emergent, urgent, acute, subacute, and chronic care with timeliness measured in seconds, minutes, hours, days, weeks, months, and years, depending on the urgency of the medical condition (Table. The Spectrum of Timeliness). The first step to timely care is access to health care. Once health care is accessed, health care providers and the systems they work in need to evaluate and treat their patients in a timely fashion. In this chapter, we look at issues revolving around the timely access to health care in both the acute and chronic care settings. We then examine the effect of timely care on patients, providers, and the health care system. Finally, we look at best practices in timely care as well as consider future directions.

S. J. Harder · E. S. Chu (✉)
UT Southwestern Division of Hospital Medicine at Parkland Hospital, Department of Internal Medicine, UT Southwestern Medical Center, Dallas, TX, USA
e-mail: Stephen.Harder@utsouthwestern.edu; Eugene.Chu@utsouthwestern.edu

© Springer Nature Switzerland AG 2020
P. V. Sreeramoju et al. (eds.), *The Patient and Health Care System: Perspectives on High-Quality Care*, https://doi.org/10.1007/978-3-030-46567-4_9

The Spectrum of Timeliness in Health Care

	Seconds	Minutes	Hours	Days	Weeks	Months	Years
	Emergent	Urgent	Acute		Subacute	Chronic	
Pathology	Cardiac Arrest from Ventricular Fibrillation	Septic Shock from Acute Cholecystitis	Severe Sepsis from Acute Cholecystitis		Symptomatic Cholelithiasis	Asymptomatic Cholelithiasis	
Access	Emergency Medical Team	Hospital Emergency Dept Intensive Care Unit	Hospital Emergency Department Acute Care Ward		Urgent Care or Primary Care Clinic	Primary Care Clinic	
Evaluation	Rhythm	Blood cultures, Lactate, CVP, Arterial Blood Pressure	Blood Cultures, Lactate, Right Upper Quadrant Ultrasound		Pre-operative Evaluation	Symptom Monitoring, LFTs, Abdominal Ultrasound	
Treatment	Defibrillation	Antibiotics, Fluids, Pressors	Antibiotics, Fluid Resuscitation		Elective Cholecystectomy	Watchful Waiting	

In the case of cholelithiasis (gallstones), when asymptomatic, timely access to primary care clinics and providers facilitates the timely ordering and execution of appropriate diagnostics as well as proper oversight for watchful waiting so that if gallstones become symptomatic, progression to an elective cholecystectomy proceeds in a safe and measured manner. Or, if the gallstones never become symptomatic, patients may avoid surgery altogether. Conversely, lack of timely access, evaluation and treatment leads to presentations in more severe forms of the disease, such as acute cholecystitis which, if not diagnosed and treated promptly, can present as or evolve into severe sepsis, septic shock or even cardiac arrest. Optimizing outcomes depends upon timely access, timely evaluation and timely treatment. In the same disease entity in the same patient, how timeliness is measured depends upon the manifestation of the disease at the time of presentation to the health care system.

The State of Timeliness of Chronic Care

In 2014, misconduct allegations of preventable patient deaths within the Veterans Affairs system were brought forward. The VA Office of Inspector General (OIG) hotline received a report stating that forty patients had died while awaiting primary or specialty care within the Phoenix VA Health Care System. While the original allegation did not identify forty specific patient deaths, preliminary investigation and OIG reporting released in May 2014 did substantiate that "significant delays in access to care negatively impacted the quality of care at this medical facility" [2].

By August of 2014, the VA completed its initial investigation of patient care delays, offering a comprehensive glimpse into the systemic inefficiencies, under-staffing, and administrative work-arounds within the Phoenix system. In all, the report detailed forty-five patient cases in which patients either died while waiting to be seen, or in whom delays in medical access led to increased morbidity. It found that a majority of reviewed veteran patients were on official or unofficial wait lists and experienced delays in accessing primary and specialty care, as well as mental health services. Patients who were treated in the emergency department setting, were recently hospitalized, were temporarily seen in the VA Phoenix system, or who were seeking to establish care were identified by the report as disproportionately affected.

While the United States Department of Veterans Affairs has received national attention, concerns of the adequacy and impact of patient wait times are not unique to that system. The "Merritt Hawkins 2017 Survey of Physician Appointment Wait Times" [3] surveyed the average wait time for a Medicare or Medicaid patient to see a physician in a primary care, orthopedic, obstetrics-gynecology, dermatology, or cardiology specialty across the United States. Among the survey findings was an average 24.1 day wait time in major metropolitan areas and 32 days in midsized markets. Perhaps, most disconcerting were disproportionate delays in primary care and an average increase in wait times of 5.5 days since 2014.

As we enter the mid-twenty-first century, wait times across industries outside of health care have become increasingly diminished. Internet retail offers doorstep delivery within the hour and videos on demand have made the local video rental store obsolete. Technology has changed the public expectation and tolerance for waiting. But despite the cultural shift, prolonged medical wait times, be they on the phone, in the doctor's office, or on a hospital stretcher, seem an immutable feature of the US health care system.

The State of Timeliness of Acute Care

On July 16, 2019, in Houston, Texas, a patient died in an overcrowded hospital's emergency department's waiting room "without receiving timely treatment," the second death of a patient waiting for emergency care in the Houston hospital in under six months [4]. Only three months later, a patient dies in the waiting room of a York, Pennsylvania, emergency department while waiting for care [5].

The lack of timely diagnosis and treatment of chronic conditions often results in chronic illnesses becoming acute, urgent, or emergent medical conditions, which necessitate immediate care. Failing to prevent progression to acute, urgent, and emergent conditions increases the burden on limited acute care resources, which, at a certain point, results in the lack of an ability to diagnose and treat acute conditions in a timely fashion.

In addition to the progression or transformation of chronic medical conditions to acute ones, on a practical level, when patients do not have timely access to primary care, they naturally seek care in inappropriate settings such as urgent care centers or emergency departments (EDs). Combined with excess, preventable acute medical conditions, heavy, unmet demand for chronic care services results in ED overcrowding. In the United States, this overcrowding has grown to crisis proportions [6].

ED overcrowding has been correlated with increased patient mortality at 10 days as well as increased mortality in the ED and increased ED revisits within 72 hours of discharge from the ED [7, 8]. While the causal pathway between ED overcrowding and worsened patient outcomes has not been well defined, the lack of a right sized structural capacity to meet demands leads to delays in both diagnosis and treatment. Structural capacity refers to both the physical environment (beds, stretchers, rooms, telemetry boxes, CAT scanners, MRI machines, and IV pumps) and the staffing levels (physicians, nurses, pharmacists, therapists, transport, and technicians). Without adequate staffing, timely patient evaluation becomes a challenge. And once the evaluation is performed, the overtaxed physical environment may lead to further diagnostic and therapeutic delays.

For example, hypertension is recognized as the largest contributor to the global burden of disease and early diagnosis and treatment of hypertension lead to improved outcomes [9]. However, hypertension is controlled in less than 20% of patients worldwide, and less so in patients in low socioeconomic strata [10]. Patients with poorly controlled hypertension over long periods of time have a higher likelihood of presenting with a hypertensive crisis such as a hypertensive urgency (76%) or emergency (24%), which may require costly hospitalization in the intensive care unit setting [11, 12]. Once in the hospital, usually starting in the emergency department, prompt treatment is critical in improving morbidity and mortality. What was once a chronic condition where timeliness of diagnosis and treatment was measured in units of months to years has now become an urgent or emergent condition where timeliness is measured in units of minutes to hours [12].

The resources required in both the emergency department, inpatient wards, and intensive care unit with regard to both the personnel (physicians, nurses, pharmacists, and technicians) and the physical environment (emergency department and intensive care unit beds, CT scanners, medications, and IV pumps) stretch the health care system. Just as emergency departments are suffering from overcrowding, critical care resources do not meet demand, resulting in rationing of intensive care unit beds [13]. Accordingly, as other patients present to the emergency department and hospital with complications or progressions of chronic diseases now in acute and emergent conditions, there will be a tipping point or threshold where the capacity of the local health care environment and system can no longer keep up with demand for care, leading to further delays and a cascading of risk for patients, providers, and the health care system alike [14]. Tragically, in extreme cases, inadequate access and delays in care can lead to premature mortality as has been seen in emergency department waiting rooms around the United States [4, 5].

The Impact of Timeliness on Patients

Inappropriate and/or unnecessary delays in care, whether measured in seconds, minutes, or hours in the emergency department, or months to years in the outpatient setting, have an emotional and physical cost to patients, health care workers, and ultimately to the health care system. The inability to address these delays introduces all involved in the health care process to suboptimal outcomes and excess morbidity and mortality.

Evidence for the health cost of care delays has been expanding over the past decade. While still limited, research demonstrates that delays impact all health care settings and health care conditions ranging from hemoglobin A1C to heart disease. The importance of timeliness of care on mortality is now widely accepted in the emergency room setting. Evidence-based timeliness metrics for sepsis, pneumonia, stroke, and myocardial infarction are now standard and accepted as beneficial to patient outcomes by the medical community. As such, substantial resource has been dedicated by the health care system to improve, monitor, and ultimately rate acute care facilities on time-based metrics. Both processes and resource allocation contribute to the satisfaction of these accepted metrics and, ultimately to improvement of care. One such example is sepsis, accounting for over 5% of all hospital expenditures and associated with substantial mortality. Drawing a connection between timeliness and outcomes, the Surviving Sepsis Campaign developed widely adopted treatment bundle recommendations for 3-hour and 6-hour benchmarks based on expert consensus [15]. Going further, studies evaluating the effects of the Surviving Sepsis recommendations suggested that no delay was safe. Pruinelli et al. evaluated the casual effect and survival probabilities of time to blood cultures, lactate levels, fluid resuscitation, and antibiotic administration – all components of the 3-hour Surviving Sepsis recommendations. In each case, they found that delays increased the risk of death, even if performed within the standardized timeframe. A delay as short as 20 minutes obtaining a patient's serum lactate level statistically impacted patient mortality [15, 16]. Based on the recognition that expeditious care is paramount to patient outcomes, the 2018 Update to the Surviving Sepsis bundle consolidated prior recommendations into a "1 hour bundle" [16].

Tissue ischemia, no matter the organ, also epitomizes the time–outcome relationship. "Time is Brain" and "Time is Muscle" are recognized axioms in the medical community. Quantitative research offers good support for these phrases. In the case of acute ischemic stroke, the relationship between the time-to-revascularization and irreversible tissue loss is well established. In patients experiencing a large vessel acute ischemic stroke, 1.9 million neurons, 14 billion synapses, and 12 kilometers of myelinated fibers are destroyed each minute. Compared with normal brain aging, the ischemic brain ages 3.6 years for each hour without treatment [17]. In these cases, expedient care is the standard of care, and time-based metrics are included in Joint Commission stroke unit accreditation.

Time to treatment in the surgical context often depends on resource availability. Physician, nurse, ancillary staff, and operating room infrastructure all represent the overhead a hospital must maintain in order to supply high-quality, on-demand emergency surgical coverage. In the case of life-threatening surgical soft-tissue infections, hospitals that are capable of meeting such requirements provide more efficient door-to-operating room transitions and experience better outcomes. In 2015, a study of 1690 surveyed hospitals found that hospitals with "around-the-clock" general surgeon and recovery room nursing had decreased mortality for life-threatening surgical emergencies when compared to hospitals without continuous in-house coverage [18]. Time to treatment factors prominently in patients experiencing myocardial infarction and acute stroke, with decisions to treat, outcomes, and institutional certifications all depending on times from presentation to definitive intervention. Across the acute care spectrum, the bar for time-based performance continues to rise.

Therapeutic timeliness for chronic disease management does not draw the same focus, but literature suggests that there are meaningful consequences for the patient and cost of care. A retrospective evaluation of VA and Medicare claims data found that shorter wait times for a primary care doctor were associated with a decreased HbA1c of 0.18 percentage points for poorly controlled patients [19]. Patients who have timely referral to cardiac rehab are more likely to improve cardiopulmonary fitness, decrease body fat and resting heart rate, and complete the recommended course of therapy [20]. Data collected from across the Department of Veterans Affairs suggested that wait times of less than a month were associated with decreased odds of hospitalization and mortality as compared to patients seen later [21, 22].

Predictably, the relationship of timeliness and suboptimal patient outcomes is most pronounced in vulnerable populations. This insight is palpable to those who directly feel the frustration and pain of waiting for an appointment or surgery. While providing clinical care to an indigent patient on the inpatient setting, I once had to inform him that his urgent surgery was postponed for a second time. He shrugged, poignantly commenting that "A person can pay for their care with time or with money. I don't have any money, so I guess I will wait." Age, economics, race, location, function, and myriad other factors impact a patient's exposure to long wait times and worsened outcomes. Elderly adults seen in facilities with average wait time >30 days were 21% more likely to die in a six-month period [22]. A number of analyses utilizing the United States National Cancer Institute's Surveillance, Epidemiology and End Results (SEER) cancer registry reported increased treatment delays for breast cancer for black women compared to white women [23], delays in initiation of adjuvant chemotherapy for rural patients [24], and increased time to therapy for colorectal cancer chemotherapy in older patients or those with multiple comorbidities [25]. In a medical profession that prides itself on recognizing the equality of humanity, disparities in timeliness hide the best of intentions and subject vulnerable patients to a lesser standard of care.

Patient experience has become an increasingly important outcome to patient care. No matter the medical, socioeconomic, or cultural background of a patient, the need to feel confidence and satisfaction in the patient–physician relationship exists. Such a confidence inspires trust and ultimately contributes to the mental and physical well-being of the patient and health care provider. The patient–physician encounter, by its nature, may also be anxiety-provoking and emotionally charged, and the effect of waiting for care only serves to exacerbate the condition. The concept of timeliness and its impact on patient satisfaction has been ingrained in most medical institutions over the past several decades, so much so that hospital reimbursements are now tied to survey results and health care organization websites frequently advertise real-time wait times at the local emergency room. These organizations realize that horror stories of long waits on the internet and by word-of-mouth can impact the bottom line.

The correlation of wait times and patient satisfaction is not difficult to conceptualize. The waste of time, as a limited resource, impacts each person in a tangible way. Altarum, a nonprofit research and consulting firm, evaluated the cost of travel and waiting from 2006 to 2017 based on the Bureau of Labor Statistics' American Time Use Survey [26]. The survey found that travel and waiting accounted for more than 50% of the time spent actually receiving medical care. Quantified using individual wages, the financial impact averaged $89 billion dollars annually. This impact was over twice the length of the next closest industry. The financial, physical, and personal opportunity costs of medical care delays are acutely felt by each patient differently, but tangibly.

Emergency departments have been at the forefront of wait time reductions, largely because the "time to be seen" has been shown to be a major driver of satisfaction in that setting. The "Golden Hour" concept, made famous in the trauma surgery arena, is now also frequently applied to the emergency department. This is not without reason. Institutional studies have shown that patient tolerance for waiting dramatically decreases after the first hour and this waiting can drive not only decreased satisfaction, but also decreased confidence in the provider and the perceived quality of care [27]. The effect is dose-dependent, with longer waits contributing to incremental detriments. Growing empirical and strong experiential evidence suggests that this same phenomenon applies to ambulatory settings, hospitals, home-based services, and procedural suites, just about any venue where the patient interfaces with the health care system. Especially concerning, a lack of timeliness which drives a negative perception of health care quality may actually be a self-fulfilling prophecy, with patients exhibiting less compliance with prescribed therapy and follow-up and predictably worse clinical outcomes [28].

In the end, the waiting patient doubly suffers.

The Impact of Timeliness on Providers

The impact of timeliness, or the lack thereof, may also impact the clinician. At the individual level, physicians and medical staff ubiquitously have first-hand knowledge of the effect health care delays have. The expression of empathy by providers for waiting patients may manifest in myriad ways – some work overtime to accommodate more patients, some step forward to lead process improvement. Most offer heartfelt apologies and internalize a system-produced harm, the accumulation of which can have a significant long-term negative impact on professional well-being.

As noted earlier this chapter, long wait times are commonplace across the health care continuum and impact providers in every setting. In outpatient clinics, long wait times ultimately contribute to patient discouragement and increased "no-shows" rates, prompting a filling of vacancies by a reactionary "double booking" of urgent patients and commonplace patient "surges." Emergency rooms and acute care settings operating near full capacity feel enormous pressure to stretch resources, including that of the provider treatment team. The chronic impact of high patient volumes, and the accompanying excess fatigue, has been associated with increased medical error. For nurses, cross-sectional analysis has demonstrated a significant association between patient mortality and low staffing [29]. Physicians self-identify a similar trend. In a study of almost 900 hospital medicine physicians, Michtalik and colleagues found that 40% of physicians reported an inpatient census that exceeded safe levels at least monthly; 36% of these reported a frequency of greater than once per week [30]. Adverse patient events generated by high census and fatigue levels may be especially impactful on clinicians, resulting in "second victim symptoms" of guilt, hypervigilance, and self-doubt that impact both personal well-being and professional functioning [31].

Many physicians will intellectualize a relationship between limited medical resources and high clinical demand, yet minimize its real-time personal impact until a critical impasse is reached. Already working most evenings and weekends to finish charting and follow-up on results, the point is reached where working harder and longer becomes untenable. Physicians, trained in a culture to prioritize their patients and their professions above their own well-being, expect to work hours beyond the traditional work week. Arndt and colleagues found that primary care physicians spend nearly an hour and a half daily working in the electronic health records after hours, known as "pajama time" [32]. One recent opinion editorial in the New York Times suggests that "the business of health care depends on exploiting doctors and nurses" [33]. As Dr. Ofri notes, "If doctors and nurses clocked out when their paid hours were finished, the effect on patients would be calamitous." In essence, physicians and nurses realize that timely care is good care. Unlike many other workplaces, in health care, many things cannot just wait until tomorrow (or even until the next hour). The hidden curriculum in medical education can be thought of as the informal teachings, often through demonstrated behaviors and attitudes of faculty physicians, which creates a gap between what is being overtly taught and what is being actually learned [34]. Accordingly, one of the hidden curricula of physician training is dedication to patient and profession as exemplified by the overt teaching about wellness and self-care and the demonstrated behaviors of overwork and working while sick [35].

This socialization of professional culture, when merged with systems of care where demand for physician services outstrips supply and the knowledge that timely care is a key contributing factor to appropriate outcomes, compels physicians to work beyond their expected hours and well into pajama and personal time. As one might expect, physician burnout has become an epidemic with Rotenstein and colleagues finding an overall prevalence of 67% in their systematic review of physician burnout [36]. Similarly, nursing burnout is highly prevalent with upwards of 40% of nurses experiencing burnout [37]. The prevalence of physician and nursing burnout far outstrips the burnout rates of the general population [38].

The Impact of Timeliness on the Health Care System

Delays in care not only adversely impact patients and providers, they also increase costs to the health care system as a whole, limiting its ability to provide care with limited health care dollars, and, in a vicious cycle, further exacerbating delays and the costs due to lack of timely care. In their June 2017 New England Journal of Medicine Perspective report, Dr. Ryu and Dr. Lee observed that just as longer wait times increased revenue for physician offices and hospitals, they increased the overall cost of health care for health care systems [39]. Based on the Geisinger Health Plan experience, they found that utilization of emergency services was 8.7 times higher for patients awaiting appointments. Adjusting for confounders, it was estimated that for every 5- to 8-day reduction in outpatient appointment waiting times, Geisinger would experience a $1 to $2 million reduction in cost.

Perhaps an unintended excess cost to delays in care is the cost of burnout that providers working in a backlogged system experience. Han and colleagues found that physician burnout costs the United States health care system approximately $4.6 billion annually. From the nursing perspective, while total costs of burnout on the United States health care system are unknown, Cimiotti and colleagues found that hospitals in which nursing burnout was reduced by 30% had a total of 6239 fewer infections, for an annual cost saving of up to $68 million [40]. Total costs of nursing burnout are likely far greater and may approach those associated with physician burnout.

Improving Timeliness of Care

As we have seen, improving the timeliness of care can have beneficial effects on patients, providers, and the health care system alike. To improve the timeliness of care, the two major avenues for health systems engineering include creating the structures which allow for proper, timely access to health care providers and facilities and the processes which allow those provider and facilities to operate efficiently and reliably.

On a health systems level, having adequate facilities and staffing to provide timely care improves health outcomes of the neighborhood, community, town, city, state, or nation it serves. Having a proper ratio of outpatient clinics and providers as well as funding for patients to access those resources will reduce unnecessary use of emergency departments and acute care hospitals. Similarly, having enough primary care providers and support staff will allow the provision of good chronic disease management and preventive care services that prevent progression and transformation to acute, urgent, and emergent medical conditions from happening. In the outpatient setting, a good measure for access is the third-next-available appointment – defined as the wait time for the third appointment available for a new patient evaluation, routine exam, or follow-up appointment. The third-next-available appointment is a more sensitive measure of outpatient access, as it accounts for random cancellations or no shows that affect first available appointment measures. The Institute for Health Care Improvement advocates for a same-day third-next-available appointment for primary care and a two-day third-next-available appointment for specialty care [41].

In the acute care setting, staffing the hospital with adequate physicians for the services that are demanded will allow for timely evaluation. Adequate beds, whether in the emergency department, intensive care units, telemetry floors, progressive or step-down units, as well as routine medical and surgical floors, are also indicated. And as beds increase, proportional increases in ancillary services such as imaging, laboratory, and pathology are required. Vizient® has started to track median time of ED arrival to transfer to inpatient unit for admitted patients as well as median time from arrival to discharge for patients discharged from the ED [42]. Once in the hospital, timely admission orders and evaluation by inpatient physicians and nurses are metrics that would inform quality of care.

With limitations on physician supply as well as financial constraints, role appropriateness should be considered in properly staffing facilities whether ambulatory clinics or acute care hospitals. A team of advanced practice providers, nurses, pharmacists, clerical staff, and technicians built to work seamlessly with physicians should improve access and timeliness of care while optimally leveraging health care dollars.

Once able to access health care facilities and providers, health care systems and processes should also support reliable and accurate delivery of health care. Missed or incorrect diagnoses result in delays in treatment and can obviate the good done by building the proper capacity of health care facilities and providers.

Future Directions

The last decade has seen a rapid expansion in technology and products in health care. But as this chapter has illustrated, access to health care, both in the acute and chronic settings, has left a greater proportion of the US population with less access, resulting in longer wait times and worsening outcomes. Indeed, between 2014 and 2017, the average life expectancy in the United States dropped for three consecutive years, despite medical breakthroughs and the highest per capita spending on health care in the world [43].

In the near to medium-term, improving outcomes in the United States will depend heavily on improving access to care. Policy decisions at the federal and state levels have a tremendous impact on the rate of uninsured persons. The expansion of individual health care funding through the Affordable Care Act (ACA) has provided many with greater access to timely diagnosis and treatment of their health care conditions. Indeed, according to the United States Census Bureau, the uninsured rate fell from 16.6% in 2013 (pre-ACA) to 10.4% in 2016 [44]. The uninsured rate in 2017 and 2018 increased to 10.7% and 11.1%, respectively, reflecting the impact of federal executive policy on population access to health care. Future lawmaker decisions in structuring the health care insurance and delivery system will feature prominently in access to timely health care and improved outcomes for Americans.

Information innovations and changing the venues of health care delivery also have the potential to provide greater access with fewer resources. The advent of stand-alone urgent and emergent care facilities in the community is one example, potentially improving access to care and relieving pressure on hospital-incorporated Emergency Departments. The impact of freestanding emergency facilities is not yet well understood, but a study evaluating utilization in Texas from 2012 to 2015 found that visitations increased 236% and another analysis found that hospital-based ED utilization increases when freestanding facilities are closed [45, 46]. Thus, expansion of this acute care setting may have a positive future impact on community access to acute care. Innovations in telehealth and electronic consults also serve to provide more timely access to primary, specialty, and even critical care. By bringing the physician to the patient and eliminating transportation times, physician resources are maximized and patient wait times are minimized. Even in the complex ICU setting, preliminary data suggests that adoption of telemedicine results in outcomes that are at least equivalent to standard care while improving access using the telemedicine model [47]. Electronic consults, asynchronous consultative provider–provider communications within the electronic health record, are another novel innovation that may improve primary provider access to specialty care and extend the impact of limited subspecialty services. Again, federal policy and reimbursement regarding both telemedicine and electronic consults are evolving, but essential in defining the future direction of remote access to timely care.

Advanced medical informatics, especially in the age of further refined electronic health record systems, may also be critical to improving resource utilization. Information sharing and avoidance of duplicity within the health care system improve access by freeing up personnel and equipment, allowing more patients to be served in a timely manner. Integration of health record sharing and systems to assist physicians in evidence-based ordering are both evolving, but hold great promise in improving utilization of existing resources and getting the most impactful studies to the right patient at the right time.

The human factor also features prominently in the future of timely health care delivery. Medical professionals, on the whole, are hard-working and selfless individuals. The health care system has long relied on their resilience and increased sacrifice to handle increased patient volume. Data on timely health care delivery would suggest, however, that the US health care system is at a tipping point, with the supply of patients outstripping the demand for providers. Future attention by federal, state, and local governments to increased training of medical personnel, as well as policies to promote increased time with patients and reduced administrative burden and burnout, will be necessary to meet the growing demand for timely care by an expanding and aging US population.

Conclusions

Timely care is an essential dimension of quality. Lack of timely diagnosis and treatment of chronic medical conditions can result in chronic medical conditions progressing and/ or transforming to acute, urgent, or emergent medical illnesses. These preventable acute illnesses tax the limited supply of acute care facilities and providers, leading to further delays and adverse outcomes of care. Taking measures to ensure timely care provides downstream benefits for patients, providers, and the health care system alike.

References

1. Institute of Medicine (US) Committee on Quality of Health Care in America. Crossing the quality chasm: a new health system for the 21st century [Internet]. Washington, D. C: National Academies Press (US); 2001 [cited 2020 Feb 27]. 360 p. Available from: https://www.ncbi. nlm.nih.gov/books/NBK222271/.
2. Department of Veteran Affairs (US). Veterans Health Administration Interim Report: review of patient wait times, scheduling practices, and alleged patient deaths at the Phoenix Heath Care System. Phoenix: VA Office of Inspector General; 2014. 28 p. Report No.: 14-02603-178.
3. Hawkins M. 2017 survey of physician appointment wait times and Medicare and Medicaid acceptance rates [Internet]. Dallas: Merritt Hawkins; 2017. [cited 2020 Feb 27]. Available from: https://www.merritthawkins.com/uploadedFiles/MerrittHawkins/Content/Pdf/mha2017wait-timesurveyPDF.pdf.
4. Ackerman T. Another patient dies in Ben Taub ER waiting area. Houston Chronicle [Internet]. 2019 [cited 2020 Feb 27]. Available from: https://www.houstonchronicle.com/news/health/ article/Another-patient-dies-in-Ben-Taub-ER-waiting-area-14189332.php.
5. Stallsmith, S. Dying patient was in ER for hours, hospital delayed reporting death, officials say. USA Today [Internet]. 2019 [cited 2020 Feb 27]. Available from: https://www.usatoday.com/story/ news/nation/2019/10/12/er-death-report-dying-patient-pennsylvania-er-hours/3957828002/.
6. Trzeciak S, Rivers EP. Emergency department overcrowding in the United States: an emerging threat to patient safety and public health. Emerg Med J [Internet]. 2003 [cited 2020 Feb 27];20(5):402–405. Available from: https://emj.bmj.com/content/20/5/402.long.
7. Richardson, DB. Increase in patient mortality at 10 days associated with emergency department overcrowding. Med J Aust [Internet]. 2006 [cited 2020 Feb 27];184(5): 213–6. Available from: https://onlinelibrary.wiley.com/doi/abs/10.5694/j.1326-5377.2006.tb00204.x.
8. Miró O, Antonio MT, Jiménez S, De Dios A, Sánchez M, Borrás A, et al. Decreased health care quality associated with emergency department overcrowding. Eur J Emerg Med [Internet]. 1999 [cited 2020 Feb 27];6(2):105–7. Available from: https://www.ncbi.nlm.nih.gov/ pubmed/10461551.
9. Dzau VJ, Balatbat CA. Future of hypertension. Hypertension. 2019;74(3):450–7. https://doi. org/10.1161/HYPERTENSIONAHA.119.13437.
10. Egan BM, Kjeldsen SE, Grassi G, Esler M, Mancia G. The global burden of hypertension exceeds 1.4 billion people. J Hypertens. 2019;37(6):1148–53. https://doi.org/10.1097/ HJH.0000000000002021.
11. Vilela-Martin J, Vaz-de-Melo RO, Kuniyoshi CH, Abdo AN, Yugar-Toledo JC. Hypertensive crisis: clinical–epidemiological profile. Hypertens Res. 2011;34(3):367–71. https://doi. org/10.1038/hr.2010.245.
12. Papadopoulos DP, Mourouzis I, Thomopoulos C, Makris T, Papademetriou V. Hypertension crisis. Blood Press. 2010;19(6):328–36. https://doi.org/10.3109/08037051.2010.488052.
13. Orsini J, Blaak C, Yeh A, Fonseca X, Helm T, Butala A, Morante J. Triage of patients consulted for ICU admission during times of ICU-bed shortage. J Clin Med Res. 2014;6(6):463–8. https://doi.org/10.14740/jocmr1939w.

14. Gladwell M. The tipping point: how little things can make a big difference. Boston: Little, Brown and Company; 2000. 304 p.

15. Levy MM, Evans LE, Rhodes A. The surviving sepsis campaign bundle: 2018 update. Intensive Care Med. 2018;44(6):925–8. https://doi.org/10.1007/s00134-018-5085-0.

16. Pruinelli L, Westra BL, Yadav P, Hoff A, Steinbach M, Kumar V, et al. Delay within the 3-hour surviving sepsis campaign guideline on mortality for patients with severe sepsis and septic shock. Crit Care Med. 2018;46(4):500–5. https://doi.org/10.1097/CCM.0000000000002949.

17. Saver JL. Time is brain – quantified. Stroke [Internet]. 2006 [cited 2020 Feb 27];37(1):263–6. Available from: https://www.ahajournals.org/doi/full/10.1161/01.str.0000196957.55928.ab

18. Daniel VT, Rushing AP, Ingraham AM, Ricci KB, Paredes AZ, Diaz A, et al. Association between operating room access and mortality for life-threatening general surgery emergencies. J Trauma Acute Care Surg. 2019;87(1):35–42. https://doi.org/10.1097/TA.0000000000002267.

19. Prentice JC, Fincke BG, Miller DR, Pizer SD. Outpatient wait time and diabetes care quality improvement. Am J Magan Care [Internet]. 2011 [cited 2020 Feb 27];17(2):e43–54. Available from: https://www.ajmc.com/journals/issue/2011/2011-2-vol17-n2/ajmc_11feb_prenticewebx_e43to54

20. Marzolini S, Blanchard C, Alter DA, Grace SL, Oh PI. Delays in referral and enrolment are associated with mitigated benefits of cardiac rehabilitation after coronary artery bypass burgery. Circ Cardiovasc Qual Outcomes [Internet]. 2015 [cited 2020 Feb 27];8(6):608–20. Available from: https://www.ahajournals.org/doi/full/10.1161/CIRCOUTCOMES.115.001751

21. Prentice JC, Pizer SD. Delayed access to health care and mortality. Health Serv Res. 2007;42(2):644–62. https://doi.org/10.1111/j.1475-6773.2006.00626.x.

22. Prentice JC, Pizer SD. Waiting times and hospitalizations for ambulatory care sensitive conditions. Health Serv Outcomes Res Method [Internet].2008 [cited 2020 Feb 27];8(1):1–18. Available from: https://link.springer.com/article/10.1007/s10742-007-0024-5.

23. Gorin SS, Heck JE, Cheng B, Smith SJ. Delays in breast cancer diagnosis and treatment by racial/ethnic group. Arch Intern Med [Internet]. 2006 [cited 2020 Feb 27];166(20):2244–52. Available from: https://jamanetwork.com/journals/jamainternalmedicine/fullarticle/411230.

24. Hershman DL, Wang X, McBride R, Jacobson JS, Grann VR, Neugut AI. Delay of adjuvant chemotherapy initiation following breast cancer surgery among elderly women. Breast Cancer Res Treat [Internet]. 2006 [cited 2020 Feb 27];99(3):313–21. Available from: https://link.springer.com/article/10.1007%2Fs10549-006-9206-z.

25. Hershman DL, Wang X, McBride R, Jacobson JS, Grann VR, Neugut AI. Timing of adjuvant chemotherapy initiation after surgery for stage III colon cancer. Cancer [Internet]. 2006 [cited 2020 Feb 27];107(11):2581–8. Available from: https://acsjournals.onlinelibrary.wiley.com/doi/full/10.1002/cncr.22316.

26. Rhyan CN. Travel and wait times are longest for health care services and result in an annual opportunity cost of $89 billion [Internet]. Ann Arbor: Altarum; 2019. [cited 2020 Feb 27]. Available from: https://altarum.org/travel-and-wait.

27. Bleustein C, Rothschild DB, Valen A, Valatis E, Schweitzer L, Jones R. Wait times, patient satisfaction scores, and the perception of care. Am J Manag Care [Internet]. 2014 [cited 2020 Feb 27];20(5):393–400. Available from: https://www.ajmc.com/journals/issue/2014/2014-vol20-n5/wait-times-patient-satisfaction-scores-and-the-perception-of-care.

28. Dubina MR, O'Neill JL, Feldman SR. Effect of patient satisfaction on outcomes of care. Expert Rev Pharmacoecon Res [Internet]. 2009 [cited 2020 Feb 27];9(5):393–5. Available from: https://www.tandfonline.com/doi/full/10.1586/erp.09.45.

29. Needleman J, Buerhaus P, Pankratz VS, Leibson CL, Stevens SR, Harris M. Nurse staffing and inpatient hospital mortality. N Engl J Med. 2011;364(11):1037–45. https://doi.org/10.1056/NEJMsa1001025.

30. Michtalik HJ, Yeh HC, Pronovost PJ, Brotman DJ. Impact of attending physician workload on patient care: a survey of hospitalists. JAMA Intern Med. 2013;173(5):375–7. https://doi.org/10.1001/jamainternmed.2013.1864.

31. Vanhaecht K, Seys D, Schouten L, Bruyneel L, Coeckelberghs E, Panella M, et al. Duration of second victim symptoms in the aftermath of a patient safety incident and associated with the level of patient harm: a cross-sectional study in the Netherlands. BMJ Open [Internet].

2019 [cited 2020 Feb 27];9:e029923. Available from: https://bmjopen.bmj.com/content/9/7/e029923.

32. Arndt BG, Beasley JW, Watkinson MD, Temte JL, Tuan WJ, Sinsky CA, et al. Tethered to the EHR: primary care physician workload assessment using EHR event log data and time-motion observations. Ann Fam Med. 2017;15(5):419–26. https://doi.org/10.1370/afm.2121.

33. Ofri D. The business of health care depends on exploiting doctors and nurses. The New York Times [Internet]. 2019 Jun 8 [cited 2020 Feb 27]. Available from: https://www.nytimes.com/2019/06/08/opinion/sunday/hospitals-doctors-nurses-burnout.html.

34. Rajput V, Mookerjee A, Cagande C. The contemporary hidden curriculum in medical education. MedEdPublish [Internet]. 2017 [cited 2020 Feb 27];6(3):41. Available from: https://www.mededpublish.org/manuscripts/1193.

35. AAMC [Internet]. Washington DC: AAMC; [date unknown]. Navigating the hidden curriculum in medical school; 2019 [cited 2020 Feb 27]; [about 4 screens]. Available from: https://www.aamc.org/news-insights/navigating-hidden-curriculum-medical-school.

36. Rotenstein LS, Torre M, Ramos MA, Rosales RC, Guille C, Sen S, et al. Prevalence of burnout among physicians: a systematic review. JAMA. 2018;320(11):1131–50. https://doi.org/10.1001/jama.2018.12777.

37. McHugh MD, Kutney-Lee A, Cimiotti JP, Sloane DM, Aiken LH. Nurses' widespread job dissatisfaction, burnout, and frustration with health benefits signal problems for patient care. Health Aff (Millwood). 2011;30(2):202–10. https://doi.org/10.1377/hlthaff.2010.0100.

38. Shanafelt TD, Hasan O, Dyrbye LN, Sinsky C, Satele D, Sloan J, et al. Changes in burnout and satisfaction with work-life balance in physicians and the general US working population between 2011 and 2014. Mayo Clin Proc. 2015;90(12):1600–13. https://doi.org/10.1016/j.mayocp.2015.08.023.

39. Ryu J, Lee TH. The waiting game – why providers may fail to reduce waiting times. N Engl J Med. 2017;376(24):2309–11. https://doi.org/10.1056/NEJMp1704478.

40. Cimiotti JP, Aiken LH, Sloane DM, Wu ES. Nurse staffing, burnout, and health care–associated infection. Am J Infect Control. 2012;40(6):486–90. https://doi.org/10.1016/j.ajic.2012.02.029.

41. Institute for Healthcare Improvement [Internet]. Boston: IHI; [date unknown]. Third next available appointment; [cited 2020 Feb 27]; [about 2 screens]. Available from: http://www.ihi.org/resources/Pages/Measures/ThirdNextAvailableAppointment.aspx.

42. White C. The future awakens: a report on the 2016 Vizient clinical connections summit. Am J Med Qual. 2017;32(1_suppl):3S–30S. https://doi.org/10.1177/1062860617701070.

43. Woolf SH, Schoomaker H. Life expectancy and mortality rates in the United States, 1959-2017. JAMA. 2019;322(20):1996–2016. https://doi.org/10.1001/jama.2019.16932.

44. Sawyer RC, Velez D, Weister T. 2018 American community survey single-year estimates [Internet]. Washington DC: United States Census Bureau; 2019. [cited 2020 Feb 27]. Available from: https://www.census.gov/newsroom/press-kits/2019/acs-1year.html.

45. Ho V, Metcalfe L, Dark C, Vu L, Weber E, Shelton GJ, et al. Comparing utilization and costs of care in freestanding emergency departments, hospital emergency departments, and urgent care centers. Ann Emerg Med. 2017;70(6):846–857.e3. https://doi.org/10.1016/j.annemergmed.2016.12.006.

46. Allen L, Cummings JR, Hockenberry J. Urgent care centers and the demand for non-emergent emergency department visits. Cambridge, MA: The National Bureau of Economic Research; 2019 Jan. 28 p. Report No.: 25428.

47. Nassar BS, Vaughan-Sarrazin MS, Jiang L, Reisinger HS, Bonello R, Cram P. Impact of an intensive care unit telemedicine program on patient outcomes in an integrated health care system. JAMA Intern Med. 2014;174(7):1160–7. https://doi.org/10.1001/jamainternmed.2014.1503.

Effectiveness of Care

10

Stephen J. Harder and Eugene S. Chu

Introduction

Effectiveness is providing services based on scientific knowledge to all who could benefit and refraining from providing services to those not likely to benefit (avoiding underuse and overuse, respectively) [1]. At their core, health care organizations across the continuum aim to provide effective care. Examination of mission statements from any clinic, hospital, or research institution will quickly affirm this. Whether the intervention is a drug, therapy, device, diagnostic test, preventative service, or watchful waiting, the aim is to produce better outcomes for our patients. In this chapter, we will explore how the evidence for effective care is generated and perceived, the efficacy to effectiveness (E-e) gradient, how the E-e gradient is being addressed in science, and future directions in effectiveness as a dimension of quality.

The Role and Challenges of Randomized Controlled Trials and Evidence-Based Guidelines

In the modern era, best evidence primarily refers to academically focused research, with an emphasis on basic science, randomized controlled trials, and guidelines. The recognized "gold standard" for clinical evidence-based medical practice is the randomized controlled trial (RCT), which seeks to eliminate investigator bias by (1) randomly allocating subjects to two or more intervention groups to control for confounding variables and (2) blinding study participants in order to allow for the objective evaluation of data. Meta-analyses and clinical guidelines rely on RCTs to inform the individual provider seeking to provide effective treatment to the patient. Evidence

S. J. Harder · E. S. Chu (✉)
UT Southwestern Division of Hospital Medicine at Parkland Hospital, Department of Internal Medicine, UT Southwestern Medical Center, Dallas, TX, USA
e-mail: Stephen.Harder@utsouthwestern.edu; Eugene.Chu@utsouthwestern.edu

© Springer Nature Switzerland AG 2020
P. V. Sreeramoju et al. (eds.), *The Patient and Health Care System: Perspectives on High-Quality Care*, https://doi.org/10.1007/978-3-030-46567-4_10

for clinical guidelines has typically seen large, multi-centered randomized controlled trials as the highest quality of evidence, ranked above clinical evidence, with smaller, single-centered randomized controlled trials as the next tier, observational cohort and case control studies in the next tier, historical cohort or quasi-experimental studies in the next tier, uncontrolled case series below that, and expert opinion as the lowest level of evidence. Well-performed systematic reviews have more recently replaced large, randomized controlled trials as the highest quality of evidence. Taking all evidence for a particular clinical question and or outcome into consideration, recommendations in clinical guidelines are made with a strength or grade, usually in a three- or four-tiered format – strongly recommended/grade A (at least one well-conducted randomized controlled trial), recommended/grade B (observational and/or historically controlled data with generally consistent findings), weakly recommended/Grade C (observational and/or historically controlled data with generally inconsistent findings), and unresolved/Grade D (case series, expert opinion).

The Grading of Recommendations Assessment, Development and Evaluation (GRADE) now offers a transparent and structured process for developing and presenting summaries of evidence, including its quality, for systematic reviews and recommendations in health care [2]. GRADE categorizes evidence with randomized trials starting at high quality and observational studies starting at low quality. All relevant studies are considered and each outcome within each study is considered separately for quality of evidence for that outcome. If evidence from trials and studies is subject to serious or very serious risk of bias, inconsistency, indirectness, imprecision or publication bias, the evidence is scored one (serious) or two (very serious) points lower. Conversely, if evidence from trials or studies has a large effect, evidence of a gradient in dose response, or address confounding completely, the quality of evidence is modified upwards by one (dose response, confounding, large effect) or two (very large effect) points. The final rating of quality for each outcomes is rated as high, moderate, low, or very low. Overall quality of evidence is determined, including direction (for/against) and strength (strong/weak).

Evidence-based medicine has always been about finding answers to guide individual patient care. Such a wealth of data has been compiled, however, that it has become impossible for the clinician to know and apply it all at the bedside. Guidelines developed from a need to consolidate RCTs, observational trials, and expert opinion and communicate this best evidence to clinicians. The resulting recommendations inform which care is deemed necessary and appropriate for specific subsets of patients. In practice, guidelines have been used to influence practice, provide a substrate for medical education, and inform decisions about benefits coverage, medical necessity, and organizational compliance with best practice.

Clinical practice guidelines became necessary because of the untenable volume of RCTs and the challenge to clinicians to apply evidence to patient care. Over the past two decades, the production of clinical guidelines themselves has undergone proliferative growth. In 2003, totally 1402 guidelines were indexed on the National Guideline Clearinghouse (NGC). This number increased to 2619 by 2013. Establishment of rigorous methods for guideline development has since decreased this number to 1440 in 2018. These guidelines are published by organizations interested in consolidating information and making it more accessible to clinicians. In many instances, however, multiple organizations may publish differing guidelines on the same medical topic. Both the American College of Cardiology/American Heart Association (ACC/AHA) [3] and the European Society of Cardiology/European Society of Hypertension (ESC/ESH) [4] published guidelines on the management of hypertension in 2017 and 2018, respectively. Both highly respected organizations sought to address a wide variety of topics relating to the diagnosis and treatment of hypertension. In both guidelines, there was concordance on most of the recommendations, including agreement on increased use of home monitoring, improved attention to in-office blood pressure monitoring, the importance of lifestyle modifications, and a focus on improving adherence to medical therapy. These agreements served as useful signposts for primary care physicians striving to apply a vast pool of information to the individual patient. Fundamental differences, however, existed. The guidelines utilized different methodologies for calculating the 10-year cardiovascular event risk, placed substantially differing emphasis on the discussion of isolated systolic hypertension, and varied even in the definition of hypertension (>130/80 mm Hg for everyone in the ACC/AHA recommendations vs >140/90 mmHg with a goal of >130/80 mm Hg in higher risk individuals in the ESC/ESH recommendations). Both guidelines are widely recognized as high quality and offered by reputable professional organizations. At the least, however, the frontline physician is asked to make judgments based on conflicting data. At its limit, conflicting guidelines influenced by bias, interests, or incomplete data may substantially muddy clinical decision-making.

In the application of clinical guidelines, clinicians face the challenge of applying recommendations developed for a large population to an individual patient. The professional curiosity a physician demonstrates in exploring a patient's social, spiritual, cultural, and other needs is necessary to understand how generalized recommendations apply to an individual treatment. The practice of shared decision-making will be explored in later chapters. It is necessary to recognize its impact, however, during any discussion of applying evidence-based medicine to effective patient care.

Efficacy Versus Effectiveness and the E-e Gradient

Randomized controlled trials are a powerful research tool to isolate the effect of a specific therapy on a specific population. Patients, however, are not all equally responsive to the beneficial effects of a treatment, nor equally immune to harmful adverse events. In an attempt to prove that a therapy has a favorable benefit to harm profile, RCTs negate the impact routine practice exerts on a therapeutic modality. Will a physician prescribe for "off-label uses?" Is a patient likely to comply with three times a day dosing? Will socioeconomic factors inhibit a patient's access to a therapy? Myriad real-life characteristics of health care delivery may impact the true effect of a drug or intervention.

Efficacy can be defined as the performance of an intervention under ideal circumstances, whereas effectiveness equates to performance in the "real world." All clinical research, including RCTs, falls on the efficacy–effectiveness continuum. In order to be clinically relevant to the clinician, a therapy typically must succeed in both domains. Similar to the Alveolar-Arterial oxygen gradient (A-a gradient) in respiratory medicine, in evidence-based medicine, we define the difference between the efficacy and effectiveness as the Efficacy-Effectiveness evidence gradient (E-e gradient). Moving from efficacy to effectiveness and successfully bridging this gap requires a therapy to fulfill broad requirements, lest the efficacy trial overestimate an intervention's effectiveness in clinical practice.

Clinically speaking, a studied therapy must fulfill three basic requirements to minimize the efficacy-effectiveness gradient. Three "A"s are employed to minimize a therapy's E-e gradient – applicability, availability, and adhere-ability. In this sense, a therapy must be readily available to providers and patients, applicable and recommendable by a physician for an identifiable population, and it must be accepted and adhered to by the patients [5]. The following examples illustrate the challenges a given therapy may face when moving from clinical efficacy trials to the bedside:

- A therapy must be readily available to providers and patients:
  - Colon cancer is the second leading cause of cancer-related death in the United States and screening through colonoscopy or fecal immunochemical testing (FIT) is known to reduce the mortality of this disease through early detection. Colonoscopy and FIT testing, if universally adhered to as recommended by the US Preventative Services Task Force, are estimated to avert approximately 20–24 deaths per 1000 patients [6].

    Studies have demonstrated that 30–50% of eligible patients do not initiate screening, 40–60% of patients with normal screening results do not repeat screening, and over 50% of patients with abnormal screening do not follow up on evaluation. An effectiveness study by Singal et al. at Parkland Memorial Hospital in Dallas, TX identified social and financial barriers to colorectal cancer screening [7]. Mailed invitations for colorectal cancer screening and reduction of scheduling barriers were compared to "usual care." After lowering barriers to patient screening, the screening process was improved to 38% and 28% for colonoscopy and FIT testing, respectively, compared to 10.7% for usual care. Adenoma and advanced neoplasia detection rates increased from 4% in the usual care group to 5.3% in the FIT cohort and 14.3% in the colonoscopy cohort. In this way, while a substantial E-e gradient still exists, Singal and colleagues substantially narrowed the gap.
- A therapy must be applicable to an identifiable population and recommendable as the treatment of choice:
  - In 2008, the Sorafenib Hepatocellular Carcinoma Assessment Randomized Protocol (SHARP) trial [8] demonstrated the efficacy of the kinase inhibitor Sorafenib in the treatment of hepatocellular carcinoma. The multicenter, randomized, double-blind placebo-controlled trial evaluated patients with newly diagnosed hepatocellular carcinoma who were treatment naïve, were not eligible for or had failed surgical or locoregional therapies, had an ECOG score of 2 or less, were Child-Pugh liver function class A, had a life expectancy of

12 weeks or more, and had good hematologic, hepatic, and renal function. The study found an overall survival of 10.7 months with sorafenib vs 7.9 months with placebo in patients. The SHARP trial was a landmark finding, as prior chemotherapeutic modalities had proven ineffective for hepatocellular carcinoma.

Due to limited therapeutic alternatives, oncologists in clinical practice prescribe Sorafenib to patients outside the scope of the original SHARP trial. Analysis of the GIDEON investigation [7] as well as evaluation of use of Sorafenib [9, 10] in HCC patients using the Surveillance, Epidemiology, and End Results-Medicare database confirmed the SHARP trial results when applied to the narrow target population. In clinical practice, however, patients with more advanced disease received Sorafenib as well. Retroactive evaluation found that patients with Child-Pugh B and C or poor functional status were subject to a markedly inferior benefit: harm when the SHARP RCT results were generalized to a "real-life" clinical population.

- A therapy must be accepted and adhered to by the patient:
  - Human Papilloma Virus (HPV) is a sexually transmitted virus that causes anogenital disease in both males and females. Persistent viral infection is highly associated with most cancers of the cervix in females. Several large RCTs compared the quadrivalent HPV vaccination to placebo in over 17,000 females aged 15–26. After 3 years follow-up, the efficacy of the HPV vaccination for preventing cervical intraepithelial neoplasia (CIN 2 or more severe disease) was 97–100% in HPV-naïve populations and 44% in the overall population. With an absolute risk reduction of 53–56%, the number needed to treat to prevent one CIN 2 or more severe disease is between 1.79 (56% ARR) and 1.88 (53% ARR).

    The United States and Australia have had significantly different utilization of the HPV vaccination. In the United States, HPV vaccination rates have been reduced by limited access and the anti-vaccination movement. A study from Connecticut found that HPV vaccination increased from 45% to 61% between 2008 and 2011. During that same period, Connecticut saw a reduction of high-grade cervical lesions of 18% [10].

    Australia's national health care system introduced the HPV vaccination program in 2007 as a cost-free course for teenage girls. According to the Cancer Council Australia, the country has now seen a 78% vaccination completion rate for adolescent females and a concordant 77% reduction in the HPV infections most responsible for cervical disease. Australia's cervical cancer rate now ranks among the lowest in the world [11, 12].

We cannot conclude our section on the E-e gradient without touching upon two additional concepts key to minimizing the gap between efficacy trials and delivering effective health care. Translational science and implementation science have emerged as two key engines for moving efficacy into effectiveness. According to the NIH's National Center for Advancing Translational Sciences, "translation is the process of turning observations in the laboratory, clinic and community into interventions that improve the health of individuals and the public — from diagnostics and therapeutics to medical procedures and behavioral changes" [13]. The translational science spectrum includes five domains – basic research, pre-clinical research, clinical research, clinical implementation, and public health. Translating clinical research to public health via clinical implementation is the key step in translating efficacy to effectiveness and to realizing improvements in individual and public health.

Clinical implementation leads us to implementation science. Implementation science is defined as "the scientific study of methods to promote the systematic uptake of research findings and other evidence based practices into routine practice to improve the quality and effectiveness of health services and care" [14]. The three aims of implementation science are as follows: (1) describing and/or guiding the process of translating research into practice, (2) understanding and/ or explaining what influences implementation outcomes, and (3) evaluating implementation [15]. Those aims are achieved using five predominant theoretical models – process models, determinant frameworks, classical theories, implementation theories, and evaluation frameworks. Together, translational and implementation sciences bring clinical science to the bedside to optimize the effectiveness of our patients' care.

Driving Effective Care

In 2009, President Barack Obama signed The American Recovery and Reinvestment Act. Provisions of this bill recognized the need for improved effectiveness in health care and allocated $1.1 billion for Comparative Effectiveness Research (CER). CER, defined by the National Academy of Medicine (NAM) at the time, was "the generation and synthesis of evidence that compares the benefits and harms of alternative methods to prevent, diagnose, treat, and monitor a clinical condition or to improve the delivery of care. The purpose of CER is to assist consumers, clinicians, purchasers, and policymakers to make informed decisions that will improve health care at both the individual and population levels." Allocations to the National Institutes of Health, Agency for Health Research and Quality, and Office of the Secretary of the US Department of Health and Human Services under The Reinvestment Act have since stimulated proposals for CER studies, impacting stakeholders across the health care continuum with the hope of better delineating real-world clinical outcomes and costs and better defining best practice for individual clinicians, health care organizations, and payers alike.

Effectiveness, Comparative Effectiveness Research, and Pragmatism in Clinical Trials

The infusion of governmental funding, combined with a maturing recognition that RCTs maximize internal validity at the expense of external validity and clinical applicability, has provided stimulus for increased Comparative Effectiveness

Research, also known as "effectiveness" or "pragmatic" research. The concept of pragmatism has gained momentum in clinical trials since traditional trials were optimized, from participant selection to intervention delivery and choice and measurement of outcomes, to maximize benefits and minimize harms associated with interventions [16]. However, concern and evidence arose that highly controlled trials overestimated benefit and underestimated harm when study interventions were translated to real-world conditions. Pragmatic trials place increased emphasis on clinical goals, application, and decision-making to establish an intervention's external validity. And similar to real-world conditions, pragmatic trials often involve complex interventions executed by teams of providers as opposed to the one, isolated intervention delivered by the solo proivder in traditional randomized, controlled trials [16]. In "ideal" conditions, pragmatic trials allow participating providers to provide the investigated therapy to a readily identifiable and generalizable population and measure clinical outcomes under "real-world" conditions. Performed effectively, pragmatic studies hold the potential to minimize the efficacy–effectiveness gradient.

In order to accomplish the goal of applicability, pragmatic trials are often large – with the aim of identifying small treatment effect "signals" amidst the "noise" of social, biological, and clinical factors. These trials seek to enroll an unselected or minimally selected population and are implemented with minimal, simple procedures and data collection requirements. End points are selected in an effort to reflect major events important to the patient or clinician (i.e., myocardial infarction, stroke, infection rate, rehospitalization, and death).

One method to determine the degree of pragmatism in a trial is the Pragmatic-Explanatory Continuum Indicator Summary 2 (PRECIS-2) tool. The nine dimensions of PRECIS-2 felt to be most important to pragmatic trials include three dimensions in the recruitment of investigators and participants (eligibility, recruitment, and setting), three dimensions in the intervention and its delivery (organization, flexibility in delivery, and flexibility in adherence), two dimensions in the nature and analysis of outcomes (primary outcome and primary analysis), and the nature of follow-up. Eligibility, recruitment, and setting prioritize study participants who are representative of patients in usual care settings with recruitment strategies that align with this goal and settings reflective of usual care. Pragmatic trials also seek to be set in organizations and environments reflective of usual care and to have intervention delivery and adherence reflect usual care flexibility in contrast to the rigid delivery methods and adherence requirements of traditional, controlled trials. Similar to delivery and adherence, follow-up should also be reflective of usual care. Pragmatic outcomes should be directly relevant to study participants and all data should be included in analysis [16, 17].

Highlighting the difference between efficacy and pragmatism are two studies examining the effect of physical therapy on lower back pain. In the first study, Hides et al. sought to evaluate the effect of exercises aimed at rehabilitating the multifidus muscle on 1- and 3-year incidence of lower back pain [18]. Thirty-nine patients with a first episode of unilateral lower back pain of less than 3 weeks' duration were treated with a highly standardized exercise program, which isolated and strengthened the multifidus muscle. The intervention group was compared to a control group of patients that received only medication and advice to remain active. The study found, via a follow-up questionnaire, that lower back pain was significantly decreased at 1 and 3 years; however, the generalizability of the findings to real-world clinical practice may be lacking. Clinical resources may limit training therapists in the standardized exercise program. Patients diagnosed within 3 weeks of a first instance of unilateral lower back pain may be challenging to identify. Therapists may be unable to determine if a targeted multifidus muscle rehabilitation regimen would be superior to more general back strengthening exercises. For these reasons, a physical therapy practice may have difficulty applying Hides' randomized control trial conclusions to their own practice.

A pragmatic clinical trial by Ben-Ami et al. focused on treating chronic low back pain through encouragement of increased recreational play [19]. In this second study, 220 patients with chronic lower back pain were enrolled in either a program to increase recreational physical activity through encouragement and exposure to fear reduction techniques or treated with "usual physical therapy." The study examined the primary outcomes of pain, mental and physical health, and level of physical activity at 12 months and concluded that recreational play was more effective than usual therapy at reducing long-term disability. In clinical practice, this pragmatic study provides less specific guidance, but more applicability. All patients with chronic back pain were included, a less prescriptive (and by corollary, a less training-intensive) intervention was required, and the comparison group to "usual therapy" was more meaningful for a physical therapy practice. While both studies contributed to the medical literature, the second pragmatic trial more convincingly demonstrated effectiveness of a therapy in real-world practice.

The Role of Pragmatism in Medical Research

Pragmatic trials function to mediate the difference between what a researcher discovers in the clinical laboratory and what a physician and patient experience at the bedside. Routinely, these trials follow phase 3 trials which determine the theoretical benefits and risks of a given treatment and start to define the population most suited to its receipt. End points of pragmatic trials are driven by patient priorities and may include major life events such as major organ dysfunction, hospital admission, death, or quality-of-life measures. Pragmatic trials can also provide long-term safety data for unselected populations, although this can be complicated by collection delays, comorbidities, and alternative treatments in the real-world setting.

In order to more effectively apply clinical research to patient care, the concepts of internal validity and external validity should be viewed as a spectrum rather than a classification. Early phase, novel, or complex interventions necessarily feature more controlled environments to understand the mechanisms of action and theoretical benefit. Even in the absence of pragmatism, these studies can be game-changing. Many trials, however, may have elements of pragmatism that decrease internal control to improve clinical applicability. The involvement of pragmatic elements serves to strengthen the study's value to the ultimate end users, the individual practitioner, and their patients. In this way, efficacy and effectiveness trials are not discrete steps to therapeutic introduction, but rather a spectrum of techniques that every study should seek to incorporate whenever possible.

Applying Effective Evidence-Based Medicine

Pragmatic trials represent an effort to incorporate everyday clinical practice into the development of guidelines and practice recommendations. However, most of the literature guiding the treatment of major disease processes still is presented in guideline format. Through professional organizations and dissemination on the internet, many clinical guidelines are widely available. Yet, the recommendations found effective in the research setting continue to fail translation into meaningful clinical outcomes. Guideline-based heart failure management exemplifies this treatment gap. In their 2011 study, Fonarow et al. examined the application of six highly accepted heart failure guidelines to the general population. The evaluation estimated the existence of 67,996 potentially preventable deaths annually in the United States by the optimal implementation of six evidence-based therapies, thus highlighting the high rate of physician "nonadherence" to the best guideline-based evidence [20].

The lack of appropriate application of guidelines is still not a well-understood phenomenon, nor are organizational best practices to ease the clinician's decision-making and application of the best evidence. Several guideline development and implementation schemata have been proposed, with most incorporating the following elements [21]:

- Guidelines should incorporate checklists with interventions linked in space and time (i.e., at time of clinic discharge).
- Guidelines should identify barriers to implementation, and design supports to address these barriers (i.e., guideline departure from prior accepted practice, requirement of physician to learn new skills, and ambiguity on type of health care provider implementing guideline).
- Guidelines should be integrated for common coexisting conditions (i.e., collating risk assessment for common harms in the ICU).
- Guideline development teams should incorporate interdisciplinary teams (epidemiologists, implementation scientists, and systems engineers) to evaluate practice strategies.
- Guidelines should focus on systems, rather than the actions of individual clinicians.

With rising utilization of electronic health in clinical practice, clinical decision support tools have become increasingly sophisticated in incorporating guideline recommendations into the daily practice patterns of clinicians. In recognition of this trend, the National Academy of Medicine's Standards for Developing Trustworthy Clinical Practice Guidelines (2011) recommended that future guidelines be structured in format, vocabulary, and contest to foster use in computer-aided decision support (CDS) systems [22]. The expectation is that computer-aided clinical decision support, based on well-designed guidelines, will facilitate more timely and individualized preventative care, diagnostic testing, and disease management. The best practice of the design, implementation, and monitoring of CDS is not yet established. Methods of systematizing the translation of document-based guidelines to clinical decision support systems have been proposed by Shiffman et al., Tso et al., and other workgroups [23, 24].

The effectiveness of efforts to bridge the gap between published guidelines and CDS-supported clinical practice has been mixed. One example of a positive impact attributable to CDS was demonstrated in a pediatric practice by Kharbanda et al. [25]. The research group evaluated the hypertension recognition and treatment rates in 31,579 patients aged 10–17 in 20 primary care clinics in an integrated health care system. The computer-assisted cohort of physicians recognized hypertension in 54.9% of affected patients vs 21.3% of affected patients in the usual care group. Patients with hypertension in the CDS group were much more likely to be referred to dietitians or weight loss programs or have additional workup for hypertension. Another study in Ostergotland, Sweden, examined a CDS tool for stroke prevention in patients with 14,134 patients with atrial fibrillation. Compared to a "usual care" cohort, patients receiving CDS-assisted care had improved adherence to guidelines (73% vs 71.2%, preintervention baseline 70.3%). While no difference in stroke, transient ischemic attack, or systemic thromboembolism was noted, the CDS cohort did have a lower incidence of bleeding (12 per 1000 patients with atrial fibrillation who received CDS compared to 16 per 1000 patients with atrial fibrillation who received usual care, $p < 0.05$) [26].

A systematic review of the effective clinical decision support systems published in the Annals of Internal Medicine evaluated 148 randomized, controlled trials studying the effect of clinical decision support systems implemented in clinical settings. The study, examining both commercially and locally developed CDS systems, found that CDS had a generally favorable effect on prescribing practices, the ordering of clinical studies, and facilitating preventative care services. While the review found the data regarding the negative impacts on physician workflow and efficiency to be lacking, there still remains significant concern of the impact of CDS tools on physician workflow, especially since inefficiencies of the electronic health record have been identified as a primary contributor to physician burnout and dissatisfaction [27].

The application of effective evidence-based medicine remains a challenge for the individual provider. The accumulation of basic science research and observational studies and RCTs has overwhelmed the individual physician's ability to assimilate knowledge and given birth to more clinically applicable treatment guidelines and pragmatic trials. While we are drawing closer to the solution, evidence-based physicians of the future will increasingly rely on clinical decision support and other novel innovations to deliver the right care, to the right patient, at the right time.

As we move forward in health care, we will see the progress of translational and implementation science allowing us to practice more evidence-based medicine. Evidence is becoming increasingly differentiated and is transforming into the knowledge that informs precision medicine – medicine tailored to the specific genetic, social, and environmental factors of each individual patient. Technological advances and data infrastructure will also grow and evolve, augmenting nascent "learning health systems," which use ongoing data feedback to drive continuous improvement through their organizations [28]. Ever-more sophisticated artificial intelligence systems built into mobile apps and digital personal assistants promise to continue to help health care providers to minimize the E-e gradient and merge the cells separating efficacy trials and effective care.

Conclusion

Translating evidence to the bedside remains a challenge in modern-day health care. While effectiveness is providing services based on scientific knowledge to all who could benefit and refraining from providing services to those not likely to benefit [1], how we generate that knowledge may lead to inherent and significant drop offs between the science and the practice of medicine. That drop off is known as the efficacy-to-effectiveness gradient. To address the E-e gradient, science has started to increasingly utilize pragmatic clinical trials – a new method of knowledge generation mirroring the real-world environment of health care. Translational and implementation science further improve the effectiveness of interventions in clinical practice. In this chapter, we explored how the evidence for effective care is traditionally generated and perceived, the efficacy-to-effectiveness (E-e) gradient, how the E-e gradient is being addressed, and future directions in effectiveness as a dimension of quality.

References

1. Institute of Medicine (US) Committee on Quality of Health Care in America. Crossing the quality chasm: a new health system for the 21st century [Internet]. Washington, DC: National Academies Press; 2001 [cited 2020 Feb 27]. 360 p. Available from: https://www.ncbi.nlm.nih. gov/books/NBK222271/.
2. Guyatt G, Oxman A, Akl EA, Kunz R, Vist G, Brozek J, et al. GRADE guidelines: 1. Introduction—GRADE evidence profiles and summary of findings tables. J Clin Epidemiol. 2011;64(4):383–94.
3. Whelton PK, Carey RM, Aronow WS, Casey DE, Collins KJ, Himmelfarb CD, et al. 2017 ACC/AHA/AAPA/ABC/ACPM/AGS /APhA/ASH/ASPC/NMA/PCNA guideline for the prevention, detection, evaluation, and management of high blood pressure in adults: executive summary: a report of the American College of Cardiology/American Heart Association task force on clinical practice guidelines. J Am Coll Cardiol. 2018;71(19):2199–269.
4. Williams B, Mancia G, Spiering W, Agabiti Rosei A, Azizi M, Burnier M, et al. 2018 ESC/ESH guidelines for the management of arterial hypertension: the task force for the management

of arterial hypertension of the European Society of Cardiology and the European Society of Hypertension. J Hypertens. 2018;36(10):1953–2041.

5. Singal AG, Higgins PD, Waljee AK. A primer on effectiveness and efficacy trials. Clin Transl Gastroenterol. 2014;5(1):e45. Available from: https://www.ncbi.nlm.nih.gov/pmc/articles/PMC3912314/.

6. Zauber A, Knudsen A, Rutter CM, Lansdorp-Vogelaar I, Kuntz KM. Evaluating the benefits and harms of colorectal cancer screening strategies: a collaborative modeling approach. Rockville: Agency for Healthcare Research and Quality; 2015. 114 p. Report No.: 14-05203-EF-2.

7. Singal AG, Gupta S, Skinner CS, Ahn C, Santini NO, Agrawal D, et al. Effect of colonoscopy outreach vs fecal immunochemical test outreach on colorectal cancer screening completion: a randomized clinical trial. JAMA. 2017;318(9):806–15.

8. Llovet JM, Ricci S, Mazzaferro V, Hilgard P, Gane E, Blanc JF, et al. Sorafenib in advanced hepatocellular carcinoma. N Engl J Med 2008;359:378–90. Available from: https://www.nejm.org/doi/full/10.1056/nejmoa0708857.

9. Lencioni R, Kudo M, Ye SL, Bronowicki JP, Chen XP, Dagher L, et al. GIDEON (Global Investigation of therapeutic DEcisions in hepatocellular carcinoma and Of its treatment with sorafeNib): second interim analysis. Int J Clin Pract [Internet]. 2014 [cited 2020 Feb 27];68(5):609–17. Available from: https://onlinelibrary.wiley.com/doi/full/10.1111/ijcp.12352.

10. Sanoff HK, Chang Y, Lund JL, O'Neil BH, Dusetzina SB. Sorafenib effectiveness in advanced hepatocellular carcinoma. Oncologist [Internet]. 2016 [cited 2020 27 Feb];21(9):1113–20. Available from: https://theoncologist.onlinelibrary.wiley.com/doi/full/10.1634/theoncologist.2015-0478.

11. Niccolai LM, Julian PJ, Meek JI, McBride V, Hadler JL, Sosa LE. Declining rates of high grade cervical lesions in young women in Connecticut 2008–2011. Cancer Epidemiol Biomarkers Prev [Internet]. 2013 [cited 2020 27 Feb];22(8):1446–50. Available from: https://cebp.aacrjournals.org/content/22/8/1446.long.

12. Patel C, Brotherton JM, Pillsbury A, Jayasinghe S, Donovan B, Macartney K, et al. The impact of 10 years of human papillomavirus (HPV) vaccination in Australia: what additional disease burden will a nonavalent vaccine prevent? Euro Surveill [Internet]. 2018 [cited 2020 Feb 27];23(41):1700737. Available from: https://www.eurosurveillance.org/content/10.2807/1560-7917.ES.2018.23.41.1700737.

13. National Center for Advancing Translational Sciences. About translation [Internet]. Bethesda: National Institutes of Health; 2011 [updated 2020 14; cited 2020 Feb 27]. Available from: https://ncats.nih.gov/translation

14. Eccles MP, Mittman BS. Welcome to implementation science. Implement Sci [Internet]. 2006 [cited 2020 Feb 27];1(1). Available from: https://implementationscience.biomedcentral.com/articles/10.1186/1748-5908-1-1.

15. Nilsen P. Making sense of implementation theories, models and frameworks. Implement Sci [Internet]. 2015 [cited 2020 Feb 27];10(53). Available from: https://implementationscience.biomedcentral.com/articles/10.1186/s13012-015-0242-0.

16. Ford I, Norrie J. Pragmatic trials. N Engl J Med [Internet]. 2016 [cited 2020 Feb 27];375(5):454–63. Available from: https://www.nejm.org/doi/10.1056/NEJMra1510059.

17. Loudon K, Treweek S, Sullivan F, Donnan P, Thorpe KE, Zwarenstein M. The PRECIS-2 tool: designing trials that are fit for purpose. BMJ. 2015;350:–h2147.

18. Hides JA, Jull GA, Richardson CA. Long-term effects of specific stabilizing exercises for first-episode low back pain. Spine [Internet]. 2001 [cited 2020 Feb 27];26(11):E243–8. Available from: https://journals.lww.com/spinejournal/Fulltext/2001/06010/Long_Term_Effects_of_Specific_Stabilizing.4.aspx.

19. Ben-Ami N, Chodick G, Mirovsky Y, Pincus T, Shapiro Y. Increasing recreational physical activity in patients with chronic low back pain: a pragmatic controlled clinical trial. J Orthop Sports Phys Ther [Internet]. 2017 [cited 2020 Feb 27];47(2):57–66. Available from: https://www.jospt.org/doi/full/10.2519/jospt.2017.7057.

20. Fonarow GC, Yancy CW, Hernandez AF, Peterson ED, Spertus JA, Heidenreich PA. Potential impact of optimal implementation of evidence-based heart failure therapies on mortality. Am Heart J [Internet]. 2011 [cited 2020 Feb 27];161(6):1024–30. Available from: https://www.sciencedirect.com/science/article/pii/S0002870311002067?via%3Dihub.

21. Pronovost PJ. Enhancing physicians' use of clinical guidelines. JAMA [Internet]. 2013 [cited 2020 Feb 27];310(23):2501–2. Available from: https://jamanetwork.com/journals/jama/fullarticle/1787420.

22. Institute of Medicine (US) Committee on Standards for Developing Trustworthy Clinical Practice Guidelines. Clinical practice guidelines we can trust [Internet]. Washington, DC: National Academies Press; 2011 [cited 2020 Feb 27]. 290 p. Available from: https://www.ncbi.nlm.nih.gov/books/NBK209539/.

23. Tso GJ, Tu SW, Oshiro C, Martins S, Ashcraft M, Yuen KW et al. Automating guidelines for clinical decision support: knowledge engineering and implementation. AMIA Annu Symp Proc [Internet]. 2017 [cited 2020 Feb 27];2016:1189–98. Available from: https://www.ncbi.nlm.nih.gov/pmc/articles/PMC5333329/.

24. Shiffman RN, Michel G, Abdelwaheb E, Thornquist E. Bridging the guideline implementation gap: a systematic, document-centered approach to guideline implementation. J Am Med Inform Assoc [Internet]. 2004 [cited 2020 Feb 27];11(5):418–26. Available from: https://www.ncbi.nlm.nih.gov/pmc/articles/PMC516249/.

25. Kharbanda EO, Asche SE, Sinaiko AR, Ekstrom HL, Nordin JD, Sherwood NE, et al. Clinical decision support for recognition and management of hypertension: a randomized trial. pediatrics [Internet]. 2018 [cited 2020 Feb 27];141(2):e20172954. Available from: https://www.ncbi.nlm.nih.gov/pubmed/29371241.

26. Karlsson LO, Nilsson S, Bang M, Nilsson L, Charitakis E, Janzon M. A clinical decision support tool for improving adherence to guidelines on anticoagulant therapy in patients with atrial fibrillation at risk of stroke: a cluster-randomized trial in a Swedish primary care setting (the CDS-AF study). PLoS Med [Internet]. 2018 [cited 2020 Feb 27];15(3):e1002528. Available from: https://journals.plos.org/plosmedicine/article?id=10.1371/journal.pmed.1002528.

27. Gregory ME, Russo E, Singh H. Electronic health record alert-related workload as a predictor of burnout in primary care providers. Appl Clin Inform [Internet]. 2017 [cited 2020 Feb 27];8(3):686–97. Available from: https://www.ncbi.nlm.nih.gov/pmc/articles/PMC6220682/.

28. Chambers DA, Feero WG, Khoury MJ. Convergence of implementation science, precision medicine, and the learning health care system: a new model for biomedical research. JAMA [Internet]. 2016 [cited 2020 Feb 27];315(18):1941–2. Available from: https://jamanetwork.com/journals/jama/fullarticle/2520639.

Improving the Efficiency of Care

11

Briget da Graca, Neil S. Fleming, and David J. Ballard

What Is Efficiency?

In 2001, the National Academy of Medicine defined "efficiency" among its six aims for health care improvement as "avoiding waste, in particular waste of equipment, supplies, ideas, and energy" [1]. More recently, the World Health Organization defined efficiency as a measure of the quantity and/or quality of output (health outcome or service) for a given level of input (cost) [2]. This latter definition captures the broader perspective of "value" in health care, from which the greater opportunities for improving outcomes and decreasing costs (i.e., resource expenditure) come through ensuring comprehensive access to and coverage of the health care resources and services needed to prevent the development of disease and for early identification and intervention when disease does occur to reduce later demand for more resource-intensive, expensive care. As such, it better communicates the idea that, while *overall* health care costs and spending can be expected to decrease with improved efficiency, improving efficiency will likely require *increased* spending in certain areas, such as strategic investments in primary care and the amelioration of deficits related to the social determinants of health (SDOH) such as low literacy, food insecurity, and lack of transportation.

B. da Graca
Baylor Scott & White Research Institute, Dallas, TX, USA

Robbins Institute for Health Policy and Leadership, Hankamer School of Business, Baylor University, Waco, TX, USA

N. S. Fleming
Robbins Institute for Health Policy and Leadership, Hankamer School of Business, Baylor University, Waco, TX, USA

D. J. Ballard (✉)
Department of Health Policy and Management, UNC Gillings School of Public Health, The University of North Carolina at Chapel Hill, Chapel Hill, NC, USA

© Springer Nature Switzerland AG 2020
P. V. Sreeramoju et al. (eds.), *The Patient and Health Care System: Perspectives on High-Quality Care*, https://doi.org/10.1007/978-3-030-46567-4_11

The Current State of Efficiency in Health Care

While tremendous advancements in medical knowledge and innovation have been made in the past century, there is substantial doubt that society is getting the full value of the US$ 6.5 trillion spent worldwide on health care annually, and evidence suggesting that 30–50% of health care spending falls into the category of "waste" [3].

Efficiency and value are certainly not strengths of the United States' health care system. In 2016, the United States had the highest health care expenditure per capita of any country [4], but ranked 43rd in life expectancy [5] and 46th in maternal mortality [6]. Performance on other health status indicators is similarly mediocre.

Much of this inefficiency is engrained in the structure of the health care system and its reimbursement mechanisms. The United States' failure to provide universal health care coverage and access (other than treatment in the emergency department) is a significant driver of inefficiency: for the 28 million Americans lacking health insurance, there is little option but to wait until they are sick enough to need emergency care – which is not only itself expensive care to deliver, but will generally occur after the greatest opportunities to prevent the development or exacerbation of disease have already passed, leaving the patient with a burden of illness that negatively impacts their quality of life and ability to contribute to society, as well as with medical debt that they are unlikely to be able to pay off within their lifetimes [7]. The lack of universal coverage also creates substantial administrative waste: as an example, Tufts Medical Center in Boston, a lean and efficient organization, spent over $50 million on processing paperwork and chasing payments in 2018, while SickKids, a hospital of a similar size in Toronto, spent just over $1 million on similar activities, thanks to Canada's government-funded universal coverage [7].

Fragmented care and fee-for-service reimbursement function well for a health care system serving a population in which a patient's health care needs stem primarily from acute conditions and each care encounter is essentially an independent event. However, when a population's health needs are chronic, fragmented care encourages redundancy and increases risk for adverse events from poorly coordinated treatment. Fee-for-service reimbursement for providers, in turn, encourages maximum use of diagnostic procedures and highly paid interventions, while discouraging activities such as patient counseling or care coordination that are essential for long-term disease prevention and management but are poorly reimbursed or not reimbursed at all. The "moral hazard" that insurance creates for patients, protecting them from the full cost of the services provided, further encourages high utilization of expensive health care services by limiting the influence of affordability on patients' decision-making processes to the amounts of their deductibles and/ or co-pays.

Reimbursement mechanisms that pay higher rates for specialist treatment also discourage clinicians from pursuing careers in primary care, and the resulting inadequate supply of primary care clinicians makes it hard for patients to access the preventive and disease management care that promotes better health in the long term. This further traps the population and its health care system in the vicious cycle of over reliance on expensive and resource intensive settings and types of care.

In retrospect, the contributions of fragmented care and fee-for-service reimbursement to inefficiency in the health care system serving a population in which most health care needs and encounters relate to chronic conditions are obvious. However, identifying them as the U.S. population's health needs transitioned from acute to chronic was made challenging by the lack of systematic quality measurement. Despite work early in the twentieth century by Ernest Codman on the 'End Result Idea' – "merely the common-sense notion that every hospital should follow every patient it treats, long enough to determine whether or not the treatment has been successful, and then to inquire 'if not, why not?' with a view to preventing a similar failure in the future" [8] – routine measurement and reporting of quality indicators did not gain prominence until near the end of the twentieth century as competition in the health care market place increased (particularly in the form of managed care structures that use financial incentives to influence physician and patient behavior); geographic variation in use of medical services was documented, raising questions of appropriate use; and the availability of clinical and administrative databases and computing capability increased [9–13].

Even with the increased interest in and use of quality measurement, measurement of efficiency remains challenging. Most of the quality measures developed and implemented have been process of care measures, and focus on ensuring effective screening or treatment procedures are not underused in patients who would benefit from them. Health care efficiency measurement, in contrast, requires examining the relationship between the health gains of individuals and the cost of the health resources expended to achieve them [14]. Unfortunately, data on individual health gains are seldom available, other than in the broadest terms, such as survival for a certain period (rather than quality of life, or health and functional status), leaving most efficiency measures to rely on intermediate outputs, such as "number of patients treated" [14].

The Patient Protection and Affordable Care Act of 2010 (ACA) introduced several "efficiency-targeted" programs in Medicare reimbursement - including Hospital Value-Based Purchasing (HVBP), Accountable Care Organizations (ACOs), and bundled payments [15]. The HVBP Program rewards acute care hospitals with incentive payments for the quality of care they provide to Medicare patients [16, 17]. HVBP took effect in October 2012; it initially placed 1% of hospital's base payments "at risk" according to their performance on measures in two areas: (1) Clinical Processes of Care (drawn from those publicly reported for acute myocardial infarction (AMI), heart failure, pneumonia and surgical care) and (2) Patient Experience (drawn from the Hospital Consumer Assessment of Health Care Providers and Systems survey), weighted 70:30 to obtain a total performance score [16]. CMS evaluates hospitals for both *improvement* (relative to the hospital's own performance during a specified baseline period) and *achievement* (relative to the other hospitals' performance with the achievement threshold for points to be awarded set at the 50th percentile of all hospitals' performance, during the baseline period) on each measure, and uses the higher score toward the total performance score [16]. In the second year, CMS added an Outcome Measures domain containing the 30-day mortality measures for AMI, heart failure, and pneumonia [17]. Additional quality domains were added in subsequent years, and the amount at risk increased to 3% of the base payment, so that in the fiscal year 2019, the following quality domains and weights were applied to calculate the total performance score: Clinical Care (25%), Person and Community Engagement (25%), Safety (25%), and Efficiency and Cost Reduction (25%) [18]. A single measure makes up the Efficiency and Cost Reduction Domain: Medicare Spending per Beneficiary [19]. The 30-day mortality measures included in the Clinical Care domain, and the Safety measures related to hospital-acquired infections and other iatrogenic events [19], also incentivize increased efficiency by motivating improvements in the health output achieved from the episode of care, as well as avoiding the costs associated with treating iatrogenic events. HVBP is now in its seventh year, but evidence that it has improved the quality of care provided is largely lacking. While one study did find a significant reduction in one of the included mortality measures (pneumonia) [20], no similar effects were seen in the other mortality measures (acute myocardial infarction and heart failure); a second study found no significant impact on any mortality measure [21]. To date, its impact of efficiency of care has not been investigated and reported in the literature. Looking comprehensively at the impact of reimbursement mechanisms intended to improve value of care is critical because of the potential for unintended adverse consequences: For example, implementation of the Hospital Readmissions Reduction Program (another Medicare value-based purchasing program that reduces payments to hospitals with excess readmissions for specific conditions) has been found to be significantly associated with an increase in 30-day post-discharge mortality after hospitalization for heart failure and pneumonia [22], as well as potentially increasing health care disparities by disproportionately penalizing hospitals that were urban, major teaching, large, or for-profit and that treated larger shares of Medicare or socioeconomically disadvantaged patients [23].

ACOs are networks of physicians, hospitals, and other providers that share financial and medical responsibility for providing coordinated care to patients in hopes of limiting unnecessary spending [24, 25]. By 2018, there were 1011 ACOs in the United States with 1477 distinct active accountable care payment contracts with public (Medicare and Medicaid) and private payers, responsible for the care of 32.7 million individuals [26]. Most of the available evidence regarding the impact of ACOs on quality and costs of care comes from the Medicare ACO programs. The most commonly adopted Medicare ACO model is the Medicare Shared Savings Program (MSSP) Track 1, in which providers earn shared savings payments if their annual spending falls below the target budget, but are not required to repay Medicare if their spending exceeds the target [27]. In 2018, approximately 75% of Medicare ACOs participated through this model [27]. The remaining 25% of Medicare ACOs participated in models with "two-sided" risk: while these models offer larger shared savings payments than Track 1, participants are responsible for repaying a portion of any amount by which they exceed the target budget [27]. Analyses of the impact of ACOs on quality and costs of care show mixed results. Early data showed a net increase in Medicare costs resulting from shifts in patterns of care that increased imaging and testing expenditures, as well as medication use [28], while another study showed increasing savings achieved by physician-group ACOs participating in MSSP, but not by hospital-integrated ACOs [29]. ACOs that have successfully reduced costs have done so through reducing numbers of patients admitted to hospital or to a skilled nursing facility, while cost per hospitalization or admission remains unchanged [30]. They also spend significantly more proportionately than other ACOs on outpatient and physician/supplier costs [30]. Findings of proportionately similar spending reductions among high- and low-risk patients suggest that the savings achieved by MSSP ACOs have largely been through efforts to limit service use among all patients, rather than through the expected mechanism of better management of high-risk patients reducing the need for hospitalizations [31]. A recent study of commercial ACOs showed similar results, with modest improvements in outpatient process-based quality measures and slowed outpatient spending growth, but no significant impact on inpatient hospital cost, use, or quality measures [32].

Bundled payments are a third reimbursement strategy intended to promote increased value and efficiency in health care. With bundled payments, participating providers receive a predetermined target price for a particular episode of care, intended to cover all acute and post-acute care provided. Participating providers share in any savings and losses resulting from differences between the target price and their actual costs [33]. Medicare bundled payment programs have included the Comprehensive Care for Joint Replacement model (CJR), the Bundled Payments for Care Improvement Initiative (BPCI), and the Bundled Payment Care Improvement-Advanced (BPCIA).

CJR was implemented in 2016 as a mandatory bundled-payment model for hip or knee replacement in randomly selected metropolitan statistical areas. Hospitals receive bonuses or pay penalties based on Medicare spending per hip- or knee-replacement episode (hospitalization plus 90 days after discharge). In its first 2 years, CJR showed a modest reduction in spending per hip- or knee-replacement episode, driven largely by a decrease in the proportion of patients discharged to post-acute facilities, without an increase in complication rates [34].

BPCI was a voluntary program, implemented in 2013, in which participating providers selected both the patient encounter-type for which they wanted to participate (from a list of 48) and one of four bundling models, which differed by the portions of the care continuum included, payment mechanism, and minimum discount rate [35]. The two most popular models rewarded (or penalized) participants through retrospective reconciliation payments. Participants received reward payments when they completed an episode of care (hospital admission +90 days or post-acute care facility admission +90 days, depending on which model they had selected) for less than the target price, and paid a penalty when they exceeded it [35]. Although Medicare spending on the BPCI clinical episodes decreased, net Medicare spending still increased because the reconciliation payments made to participants were greater than the savings that had been achieved [36]. In the model starting at hospital admission, the source of cost reductions was similar to CJR: admission of fewer patients to post-acute care facilities and shorter stays for those that were admitted [36]. No negative impacts on mortality, readmission rates, emergency department visits, or functional status were identified [36].

BPCIA is as updated iteration of Medicare's bundled payment program. Participating organizations can choose among 33 types of inpatient encounter (for example, admissions for coronary artery bypass graft surgery, pneumonia, renal failure, or sepsis) and four types of outpatient encounter (for example, percutaneous coronary intervention, or total knee replacement). It operates under a total-cost-of-care concept, in which the total Medicare Fee for Services (FFS) spending on all items and services furnished during the 90-day period assigned for the encounter, including outlier payments, are considered part of the relevant expenditures for purposes of reconciling the target price with the cost of care provided, unless specifically excluded [37]. BPCIA was not implemented until October 2018, so data are not yet available on its impact on the value and efficiency of the health care delivered within it.

While reimbursement mechanisms that place portions of providers' payments at risk depending on the quality and cost of the care that they provide create incentives to improve quality and/or decrease costs, it remains up to the providers to develop strategies through which they can accomplish these aims. While the dominant strategy in the Medicare at-risk payment models to date appears to have been avoiding admitting patients to acute care facilities, other opportunities for improving efficiency exist. One that should not be ignored is standardization of care where unwarranted variation is identified [38]. For example, in a large multihospital system, where individual physicians may have developed their own preferences and styles for treating common conditions, such as pneumonia or heart failure, and different facilities or units may have different standard practices of varying effectiveness and cost, implementing – and encouraging use of – a system-wide standardized order set can achieve meaningful improvements in both clinical outcomes and cost. One large, not-for-profit health care system in Texas reported significant success with such an approach: using the standardized pneumonia order set to treat 2000 patients would save an additional 33 lives and avoid $766,000 in direct patient care costs [39, 40]. For heart failure, it was estimated that, for every 85 people treated using the standardized order set, one in-hospital death would be prevented [40].

"Lean Thinking" is a manufacturing approach to improving efficiency that has gained a following among health care providers seeking to identify and eliminate waste in their delivery of care [41], with a focus on inputs, flows/processes, and outputs [42]. Health care systems apply this approach to a variety of value streams – ranging from emergency department registration and throughput, to strategic sourcing, diagnostic imaging, and pre-admission testing [43] – seeking to improve different aspects of efficiency.

The Virginia Mason Medical Center in Seattle, Washington, has embraced the Lean approach enthusiastically, creating the Virginia Mason Production System (VMPS) in 2002, to adapt and apply the manufacturing-focused Toyota Production System to the health care context, and the Virginia Mason Institute in 2008 to educate leaders, providers, and frontline staff from other health care organizations in the use of Lean tools and methods [44]. The successes Virginia Mason credits to its adoption of the VMPS include the following:

- saving $11 million in planned capital investment by using space more efficiently
- reducing the time taken to report lab test results to the patient by >85%
- reducing inventory costs by $2 million through supply chain expense reduction and standardization efforts

- reducing labor expense in overtime and temporary labor by $500,000 in just 1 year
- increasing productivity by 93% in a few targeted areas by moving the most common supplies to point of use and creating kits containing frequently needed supplies
- reducing premiums for professional liability insurance by 56%

As these examples show, Lean thinking projects frequently target cost reductions. For this methodology to achieve true efficiency improvements, it must be coupled with monitoring of relevant quality measures to ensure that the same, if not better, levels of the desired health outcomes are being achieved for the lower cost. A review of the Lean health care projects reported in the peer-reviewed literature found that implementation is highly localized with small successes, and minimal evidence of sustainability [45], indicating a need for rigorous, long-term studies of the potential impact of broad-scale adoption of Lean thinking on health care efficiency.

Perceived Gaps – and Potential Solutions and Innovations

One of the biggest challenges in improving health care efficiency is the lack of timely, accessible, reliable, relevant data for quality measurement to guide improvement activities. To examine efficiency of care, data on both the desired health outcomes (survival, quality of life, health and functional status, etc.) and data on the resources and associated costs expended in delivering care are needed. Neither of these is readily available. Even for the most basic health outcome – survival – the United States has no up-to-date, inexpensive data source through which providers can track survival after an episode of care [46]. The situation for other desired health outcomes is even worse: routine collection of quality-of-life and functional status data is not a widespread practice in health care – nor does a centralized data infrastructure exist that would enable providers to track these outcomes (as general or disease-specific measures) longitudinally, independently of whether the patient continues to see them for care. While the "CDC Healthy Days" questions (an acknowledged standard for population surveillance of health-related quality of life by national and international groups) were included in the Behavioral Risk Factor Surveillance System (BRFSS) from 1993 to 2015, the National Health and Nutrition Examination Survey (NHANES) from 2000 to 2012, and the Medicare Health Outcomes Survey (HOS) of Medicare Advantage beneficiaries since 2003 [47], these surveys capture only a sample of the population and are not used to populate databases intended to enable individual patient-level tracking of outcomes.

What is needed is integration of routine assessment (and record) of quality of life and health status in a patient's medical records to allow changes in these outcomes to be tracked over time as part of the assessment of the benefits the patient has obtained from the health care services received. Instruments to collect these data have existed for decades, but their use has historically been largely relegated to discrete research projects, rather than integrated into health care delivery. For example, the EQ-5D was developed from 1987 to 1991 by the interdisciplinary five-country EuroQoL

Group as a standardized instrument to measure health-related quality of life that can be used in a wide range of health conditions and treatments [48]. This preference-based measure of health status is now widely used in clinical trials, observational studies, and other health surveys [49]. It has evolved from the three-level answer version (EQ-5D-3L) which measures 343 "health states" (each described by a unique five-digit number, in which each digit indicates which of the three responses the individual chose for each of the five questions, addressing mobility, self-care, usual activities, pain/discomfort, and anxiety/depression, respectively [50]) to the five-level answer version (EQ-5D-5L), which is able to describe 3125 health states. Health status scores (utilities) have been established from the general population to compute weights based on responses to the five questions, allowing measurement of how much patient health status changes over time, especially when some type of medical intervention has occurred [49]. These health status scores can be combined with measures of survival duration to compute quality-adjusted life years (QALY), and are especially helpful when effectiveness and cost-effectiveness are being deter-mined [51]. This approach has been used, for example, to examine intra-patient cost effectiveness by comparing pre- and post-measures of health status (both general and spine-specific) in relation to cost for scoliosis surgery patients [52]. Such endeavors have not yet made it, however, into routine assessments of patients' outcomes.

One possible barrier to widespread use of the EQ-5D in clinical practice may be the licensing fee required for its use [53]. No similar fee is required for use of PROMIS (Patient-Reported Outcomes Measurement Information System), which was developed with National Institutes of Health funding to provide a set of person-centered measures to evaluate and monitor physical, mental, and social health in adults and children, and that can be used in both the general population and patients living with chronic diseases [54]. PROMIS collects patient data in multiple catego-ries, including physical health, anxiety, depression, fatigue, sleep, social function, pain interference, and global health [55]. Although PROMIS was established as a research initiative, its role was subsequently expanded to support applications in clinical practice [56]. The electronic administration of PROMIS is particularly well suited to integration with clinical care as it incorporated computer adaptive testing to reduce response burden – i.e., items are dynamically selected for administration from an item bank based upon the respondent's previous answers, enabling 4–12 item responses to provide a high level of measurement precision [57]. It has further-more been shown capable of integration with an electronic medical record with little to no impact on registration times for patients completing the questionnaires [58]. A third option for capturing actionable data on quality of life and other outcomes that represent priorities for patients is implementation of the publicly available, disease- or population-specific standard measure sets developed by the International Consortium for Health Outcomes Measurement (ICHOM) [59]. These measure sets are constructed by condition-specific Working Groups, comprised of physicians, registry leaders, outcomes experts, and patient representatives, and include clinical measures (for example, for diabetes, glycemic control and development of chronic complications), patient-reported measures (for example, psychological well-being), health services measures (such as health care utilization or barriers to treatment access), and long-term outcomes measures (such as survival) [59]. Furthermore, these Standard Sets and their accompanying Reference Guides contain evidence-based guidance on which data to collect and at which time point for a given condition in order to consider the outcomes of treatment, and include evidence-based case-mix/adjustment variables that need to be considered when comparing outcomes across different patient groups [60].

Accurate cost data are frequently just as lacking in health care as patient outcome data. Some, but not all, health care provider organizations have cost accounting systems for recording, analyzing, and allocating cost to the individual services provided to patients (e.g., medications, procedures, tests, room, and board). Those that do not have such systems rely on rudimentary methods such as the ratio of cost to charge, which do not provide sufficiently accurate cost estimates [61]. Furthermore, neither the cost accounting nor the ratio of cost to charge methods are standardized across the organizations that utilize them [62], making comparability across organizations problematic. Additionally, the fragmented nature of the U.S. health care system can make it challenging to capture all costs over an entire cycle of care, which might involve multiple providers and facilities using (or not using) different systems of cost accounting [62]. Other challenges to obtaining accurate cost data include the confidential nature of contracted rates between payers and providers, and between providers and suppliers [63].

There has been substantial political interest recently in increasing price transparency in health care – for example, the June 24, 2019 Executive Order requiring the Secretary of Health and Human Services to propose regulations requiring hospitals to publicly post standard charge information, including charges and information based on negotiated rates and for common or shoppable items and services [64], and May 2019 Centers for Medicare & Medicaid Services (CMS) rule requiring direct-to-consumer television advertisements for prescription pharmaceuticals covered by Medicare or Medicaid to include the drug's list price [65]. However, such initiatives, while possibly increasing the data available regarding charges for or reimbursement received for care delivered, do not address the barriers to obtaining and using data on the actual costs incurred through the provision of those services. As such, no benefits in terms of our ability to meaningfully measure the efficiency of health care delivery can be expected. The innovation needed to address the lack of cost data is implementation of a standardized cost accounting system throughout the health care system.

The data challenges surrounding measurement of health care efficiency are further reflected in the lack of National Quality Forum (NQF)-endorsed measures for this domain. While the Cost and Efficiency Portfolio does contain seven endorsed measures, three capture hospital-level risk-standardized payments associated with episodes of care for particular conditions: one captures Medicare spending per beneficiary treated at the hospital, another measures a primary care provider's risk-adjusted cost-effectiveness at managing the population for which they care, a sixth is a risk adjusted measure of the frequency and intensity of services utilized to manage a provider group's patients, and the seventh is a measure of the percentage of patients transferred from one facility to another with documentation that the required information for treatment was communicated to the receiving facility in a timely manner [66]. With the possible exception of the measure of primary care providers' cost-effectiveness in managing the populations they care for, none of these measures captures the relationship between cost of delivering care and the achievement of the desired health outcome required for a meaningful measurement of efficiency.

Challenges in implementing meaningful measures of efficiency include reaching agreement on how quality and cost measures are combined in the measure, which can significantly impact the resulting relative incentive for providers to decrease costs vs increase quality [15]. Furthermore, assessments of the reliability and validity of measures linking quality and cost are largely lacking. Such assessments are urgently needed to enable health care providers to measure, monitor, and improve their efficiency.

What Would Be Ideal?

To properly manage value in health care (with which efficiency is inextricably intertwined [15]), costs and outcomes must be measured at the patient level and must encompass the entire cycle of care for the relevant medical condition (diagnosis, treatment and rehabilitation, and/or ongoing management), including the common complications and comorbidities of that medical condition [67]. Outcome measures need to cover multiple dimensions to capture the goals of health care – for example, survival, ability to function, duration of care, sustainability of recovery (thus also capturing "disutilities" such as complications, adverse events, and recurrences that may follow care) – and need to track the patient's course of care across all providers involved [67]. For cost measurement, the idea that charges billed or reimbursement paid in any way reflects the actual costs of care incurred in delivering the needed care must be challenged; likewise, the allocation of costs to procedures, services, or departments based on reimbursement rates (which are themselves based on inaccurate assumptions about the intensity of care, and are further distorted through rate negotiations with payers). Instead, costs need to be measured as how much of the resource's available capacity (e.g., time) is used in the care of a particular patient, regardless of the reimbursement received [67]. Such an approach eliminates the distortions in supply and efficiency of care that have resulted from the cross-subsidies that occur across services for which providers are generously reimbursed vs those on which they incur losses [67].

Accurately measuring actual costs incurred over the course of a patient's care is challenging. Patients follow complex paths through a fragmented delivery system, and getting the actual costs incurred along those paths requires tracking the sequence and duration of the clinical and administrative processes used along the way [67]. Such tracking would require updates to the information systems used by all the providers involved in the care path, as they are not currently designed to facilitate such tracking, nor to map asset and expense categories to patient processes. That is not to say, however, measuring actual costs is impossible; it can, for example, be achieved using time-driven activity-based costing (TDABC) [67]. This approach requires one to:

1. Obtain good estimates of a typical path (or set of paths) for a particular medical condition
2. For each step in the path, determine the following:
   (a) The practical capacity of all the resources involved

(i) For personnel, this can be calculated from three time estimates that are generally available from human resources data: total number of days the employee works per year, total number of hours per day that the employee is available for work, and the average number of hours per workday used for non-patient-related work (breaks, training, education, administrative meetings)

(ii) For equipment, this can be measured by estimating the number of days per month and hours per day the equipment can be used to determine its upper limit on practical capacity

(b) The capacity cost rates of the resources involved – including not only the full compensation (salary, payroll taxes, fringe benefits) for each person involved, but also their pro rata share of costs related to employee supervision, office space, information technology, telecommunications, etc. used in their normal course of work

(c) The time expended by each resource on the patient's care

Once these three measures have been estimated for each step in each relevant care pathway, total costs for the patient's cycle of care can be computed [67].

Implementing TDABC reveals the inaccurate assumptions regarding costs that follow from estimating them based on charges or reimbursement. For example, a charge-based cost system will allocate higher costs to the sterilization of surgical toolkits for coronary artery bypass graft surgery than for total knee replacement surgery, because charges for coronary artery bypass graft surgery are higher. However, TDABC shows that more time and expense are, in fact, incurred in sterilizing the more complex knee surgery tools [67].

Pilot tests of implementing TDABC have also revealed significant variation in the processes, tools, and equipment used by clinicians performing the same service, even within the same unit. Such discoveries can provide opportunities for informed discussions about standardization of care and limiting the use of expensive approaches or materials that do not produce demonstrably better outcomes [67].

Implementing TDABC alone will not, of course, automatically improve either the efficiency or value of health care. What it can do, however, is provide the accurate patient-level cost data needed, in combination with patient outcome data, to implement meaningful measurement and improvement of efficiency and value.

Organizing the collection of cost data around cycles of care can also inform the redesign of the health care system to align payment with value. Time-based bundled payments or payment for a total package of services in a defined patient subgroup with similar needs (e.g., healthy children, or elderly adults with multiple chronic conditions) for a specified period is the payment approach that aligns best with value [68]. It would allow evidence-based "per member per month" reimbursement levels to be established for the different patient subgroups being managed in primary care, or specialties that focus on chronic conditions, as well as defining the additional fee-for-service payments that would need to be available to reimburse treatment of acute care needs [68].

On the outcomes side of the efficiency equation, there is a substantial need both for expanded systematic collection of additional outcomes data – in particular, patient-reported outcomes addressing issues like quality of life, and physical, mental, and social functioning – as well as greater access to existing outcomes data, such as mortality, unplanned hospital admissions, and emergency department visits.

With respect to increased access to existing outcomes data, two sources that could be made eminently useful for tracking outcomes and resource utilization spring to mind. The first, addressing the most basic need for outcome measurement in health care (i.e., mortality) is the Social Security Death Master File. Until November 1, 2011, the Death Master File was a sufficiently timely and affordable source of national vital status data that hospitals and health care systems (although few if any individual physicians) could use to track post-discharge survival of their patients [46]. However, in 2011, the Social Security Administration determined that all the deaths that had been submitted by states via electronic death registration (~5% of the deaths recorded in the Death Master File at the time, and 40% – and growing – of the new deaths being reported) were state-owned data that were exempt from disclosure under the Freedom of Information Act, the mechanism through which the Death Master File became publicly accessible [46]. As such, they removed the state-owned death data already included in the Death Master File from subsequent releases, and stopped including any deaths reported via electronic death registration – rendering the publicly available Death Master File effectively defunct as a source of vital status data [46]. While other sources of vital status data do exist – for example, the National Death Index, as well as databases maintained by the individual states or vital statistics jurisdictions – these all have limitations that make them unsuitable for routine monitoring of outcomes by health care providers: for example, the National Death Index has a 12–18-month time lag, is costly to obtain, and is only available for research (not quality improvement or monitoring) purposes [46], while state-level databases, beyond the limitation of only including deaths that occurred within their jurisdiction, have varying time lags, costs, and rules about how and by whom the data can be accessed [46]. Meanwhile, the Social Security Administration's own version of the Death Master File continues to amass timely, national death data – but, by statute – can only be used for statistical and research activities conducted by federal and state agencies; verifying accuracy of information for voter registration; and matching data between the Social Security Administration records and the Department of Health and Human Services records [69]. It would seem reasonable for Congress to add the monitoring of health care outcomes to the list of allowed uses – and either allowing health care providers that can demonstrate the necessary data protections and safeguards (which should align with the similar need for protection of identifiable data already in place under the Health Insurance Portability and Accountability Act) to purchase subscriptions to the file or, if preferred, to establish a secure mechanism whereby providers can submit, in large batches, the identifiers of patients for whom they are seeking vital status data, and receive date of death information for those that have matches in the Death Master File. Any such innovation along these lines will likely remain wishful thinking for some time, however. Since the removal of the electronically submitted state-owned death data in 2011, Congress has added additional restrictions to access to even the "Limited Death Master File" that includes only the Social Security Administration-owned data that is subject to the Freedom of Information Act [70].

The second potential source of valuable outcomes data, with a little Congressional intervention, are All-Payer Claims Databases (APCDs). APCDs are State databases that include medical claims, pharmacy claims, dental claims, and eligibility and provider files collected from private and public payers [71]. APCD data are reported directly by insurers to States, usually as part of a State mandate. APCDs offer several important advantages over other data sets in terms of their capacity to produce price, resource use, and quality information [71]:

1. They include information on care for patients across care sites, capturing all encounters the patient has with the health care system – regardless of which hospitals, physician groups, or other providers are involved.
2. They include information from most private insurance companies operating in the state, which many other datasets do not.
3. They provide large sample sizes, geographic representation, and capture of longitudinal information on a wide range of individual patients.

By early 2018, 18 states had legislation mandating the creation and use of APCDs [71]. However, the data collected and the insured populations included vary widely between states, as do access requirements and limitations on use of the data [72].

The biggest limitation to state APCDs, however, is the 2016 Supreme Court decision in Gobeille v. Liberty Mutual Insurance Co that the Employee Retirement Income Security Act (ERISA) invalidates state APCD reporting requirements for self-funded employee health plans, depriving states of a substantial portion of the information on health care utilization, pricing, and quality in the state. Given that >60% of U.S. workers with employer-based health insurance are in self-funded plans [73], this is a substantial limitation. Since individuals who get their insurance through employers tend to be healthier, removing the majority of people with employer-based coverage from the database undermines the generalizability of analyses performed by creating a selection bias toward older and sicker individuals.

To realize the full potential of APCDs as sources of health care outcomes and resource utilization data, Congressional action is needed first to ensure that data for individuals covered by ERISA plans are included, and second, to either establish a nationwide APCD or to establish minimum standards for the populations and data types included in state APCDs, and the requirements for access to and limitations on use of data in the state APCDs.

Practical Ways to Improve Efficiency

The large-scale changes in outcome and cost measurement outlined above to facilitate meaningful measurement and improvement of efficiency in health care lie far beyond the scope of what most individual providers, payers, or patients can influence. There are, however, smaller, common-sense actions even individuals can take that, incrementally, could meaningfully improve efficiency and value. A few of these are suggested below for various health care stakeholders.

Patients
- Use out-of-network providers only when necessary
- Where access to multiple care settings is available, know the appropriate settings for different health needs (e.g., urgent care center vs. emergency department; eVisit vs. primary care office visit)
- Adopt healthy lifestyles – for example, adhering to diet and exercise recommendations, as well as medication regimens and other prescribed care
- Patients with health care insurance (or otherwise able to pay) should obtain preventive care as medically recommended to take a longer vs. short view of self-care
- Talk to providers about different treatment options available (shared decision-making), their costs, and likelihood of achieving desired outcomes – and be prepared to both educate and learn during such conversations

Health care providers
- Participate in ACOs, bundled payments, and other alternative payment programs that provide incentives to maximize value and efficiency
- Engage in shared decision-making with patients, taking into account both their goals of treatment and costs of care
- Implement the technology, infrastructure, and workforce needed to improve access to lower levels of care for acute nonurgent matters (e.g., eVisits with an advanced practice nurse) to keep more expensive care (e.g., physician office visit) for visits that require greater levels of care (e.g., chronic disease management)
- Empower staff such that everyone is functioning "at the top of their license."
- Participate in initiatives such as the "Choosing Wisely" campaign, which provide the tools and information needed to steer clinical decisions toward the health care services that truly benefit patients, avoiding waste
- Implement step-based care protocols that ensure affordable effective treatment options are exhausted before expensive options are tried
- Integrate physical, mental, and social care services, ensuring the benefits of clinical care are not undermined by unmet mental health needs or social determinants of health (such as lower level of literacy; distrust of health care professionals rather than community/peer based workers)

Payers
- Implement models of care which encourage limitation of the use of specialists to truly rare and complex conditions that fall outside generalists' scope of care
- Provide flexible funding in health care coverage that can be used to address social determinants of health and prevent the development or exacerbation of expensive medical conditions
- Provide incentives for providers to adopt cost accounting systems

Policymakers
- Improve overall efficiency by addressing social determinants of health (substandard housing, food insecurity, lack of transportation, low literacy, etc.)
- Ensure adequate access to and coverage of health care, so that problems can be identified and managed early, rather than when more expensive/extreme interventions and settings are required
- Provide incentives for more clinicians to become primary care providers and other generalists
- Bring prices into line with those paid in other developed nations – for example, exorbitant drug prices can be tackled from a variety of angles, including antitrust enforcement to maintain/increase competition among manufacturers, address aspects of patent laws and their enforcement that enable ever greening and product hopping to limit generic competition, and allow importation of pharmaceutical products from countries with regulatory oversight ensuring the safety and quality of the products that is equivalent to the provided by the U.S. Food and Drug Administration
- Provide funding for cost-effectiveness research – especially on a population health basis over the continuum of care – and allow this evidence to be used to guide treatment and coverage policies when determining how to allocate scarce resources

References

1. Committee on Quality Health Care in America, Institute of Medicine. Crossing the quality chasm. A new health system for the 21st century. Washington, DC: National Academy Press; 2001.
2. World Health Organization. More health for the money. Health systems financing: the path to universal coverage. Geneva: WHO Press; 2010. p. 61–84.
3. World Economic Forum. Global coalition for value in healthcare. https://www.weforum.org/projects/value-in-healthcare. Accessed 2 Aug 2019.
4. The World Bank. Current health expenditure per capita (current US$). 2019. https://data.worldbank.org/indicator/SH.XPD.CHEX.PC.CD?most_recent_value_desc=false. Accessed 30 July 2019.
5. Central Intelligence Agency. The world fact book: life expectancy at birth. https://data.worldbank.org/indicator/SH.XPD.CHEX.PC.CD?most_recent_value_desc=false. Accessed 30 July 2019.
6. Central Intelligence Agency. The world fact book: maternal mortality rate. https://www.cia.gov/library/publications/the-world-factbook/rankorder/2223rank.html. Accessed 30 July 2019.
7. Apkon M. What level of disparity in health care are we willing to tolerate? 2019. https://www.bostonglobe.com/opinion/2019/08/01/what-level-disparity-healthcare-are-willing-tolerate/YtOURY2Vt8s3EkgZU1CHMJ/story.html. Accessed 2 Aug 2019.
8. Donabedian A. The end results of health care: Ernest Codman's contribution to quality assessment and beyond. Milbank Q. 1989;67(2):233–56; discussion 257–267.
9. Epstein AM. The role of quality measurement in a competitive marketplace. Baxter Health Policy Rev. 1996;2:207–34.
10. Chassin MR, Brook RH, Park RE, et al. Variations in the use of medical and surgical services by the Medicare population. N Engl J Med. 1986;314(5):285–90.
11. Gittelsohn A. Small area variations in health care delivery. Science. 1973;182(4117):1102–8.
12. Wennberg JE, Freeman JL, Culp WJ. Are hospital services rationed in New Haven or overutilised in Boston? Lancet. 1987;1(8543):1185–9.
13. Nigam A. Changing health care quality paradigms: the rise of clinical guidelines and quality measures in American medicine. Soc Sci Med. 2012;75(11):1933–7.
14. Hollingsworth B. The measurement of efficiency and productivity of health care delivery. Health Econ. 2008;17(10):1107–28.
15. Ryan AM, Tompkins CP. Efficiency and value in healthcare: linking cost and quality measures paper. 2014. https://www.qualityforum.org/Publications/2014/11/Efficiency_and_Value_in_Healthcare__Linking_Cost_and_Quality_Measures_Paper.aspx. Accessed 30 July 2019.
16. Centers for Medicare & Medicaid Services. Frequently asked questions: hospital value-based purchasing program. 2012. http://www.cms.gov/Medicare/Quality-Initiatives-Patient-Assessment-Instruments/hospital-value-based-purchasing/Downloads/FY-2013-Program-Frequently-Asked-Questions-about-Hospital-VBP-3-9-12.pdf. Accessed 22 Jan 2014.
17. Department of Health and Human Services. Centers for Medicare and Medicaid Services. Medicare and Medicaid programs: hospital outpatient prospective payment; ambulatory surgical center payment; hospital value-based purchasing program; physician self-referral; and patient notification requirements in provider agreements. Final rule with comment period. Fed Regist. 2011;76(230):74122, 74527–74531, 74543–74544.
18. Centers for Medicare and Medicaid Services. Hospital value-based purchasing. https://www.cms.gov/Medicare/Quality-Initiatives-Patient-Assessment-Instruments/HospitalQualityInits/Hospital-Value-Based-Purchasing-.html. Accessed 30 July 2019.
19. QualityNet. Fiscal years 2018–2024 measures: hospital value-based purchasing. http://www.qualitynet.org/dcs/ContentServer?c=Page&pagename=QnetPublic%2FPage%2FQnetTier3&cid=1228775522697. Accessed 30 July 2019.

20. Ryan AM, Krinsky S, Maurer KA, Dimick JB. Changes in hospital quality associated with hospital value-based purchasing. N Engl J Med. 2017;376(24):2358–66.

21. Figueroa JF, Tsugawa Y, Zheng J, Orav EJ, Jha AK. Association between the value-based purchasing pay for performance program and patient mortality in US hospitals: observational study. BMJ. 2016;353:i2214.

22. Wadhera RK, Joynt Maddox KE, Wasfy JH, Haneuse S, Shen C, Yeh RW. Association of the Hospital Readmissions Reduction Program with mortality among Medicare beneficiaries hospitalized for heart failure, acute myocardial infarction, and pneumonia. JAMA. 2018;320(24):2542–52.

23. Thompson MP, Waters TM, Kaplan CM, Cao Y, Bazzoli GJ. Most hospitals received annual penalties for excess readmissions, but some fared better than others. Health Aff (Millwood). 2017;36(5):893–901.

24. Gold J. Accountable care organizations, explained. 2015. https://khn.org/news/aco-accountable-care-organization-faq/. Accessed 29 July 2019.

25. Centers for Medicare and Medicaid Services. Accountable Care Organizations (ACOs). https://www.cms.gov/Medicare/Medicare-Fee-for-Service-Payment/ACO/. Accessed 29 July 2019.

26. Muhlestein D, Saunders RS, Richards R, McClellan MB. Recent Progress in the value journey: growth of ACOs and value-based payment models in 2018. Health Affairs Blog. 2018. https://www.healthaffairs.org/do/10.1377/hblog20180810.481968/full/. Accessed 29 July 2019.

27. Mechanic R, Perloff J, Litton T, Edwards K, Muhlestein D. The 2018 annual ACO survey: examining the risk contracting landscape. 2019. https://www.healthaffairs.org/do/10.1377/hblog20190422.181228/full/. Accessed 29 July 2019.

28. Kury FSP, Baik SH, McDonald CJ. Analysis of healthcare cost and utilization in the first two years of the Medicare shared savings program using big data from the CMS enclave. AMIA Annu Symp Proc. 2016;2016:724–33.

29. McWilliams JM, Hatfield LA, Landon BE, Hamed P, Chernew ME. Medicare spending after 3 years of the Medicare shared savings program. N Engl J Med. 2018;379(12):1139–49.

30. Schulz J, DeCamp M, Berkowitz ASA. Spending patterns among Medicare ACOs that have reduced costs. J Healthc Manag. 2018;63(6):374–81.

31. McWilliams JM, Chernew ME, Landon BE. Medicare ACO program savings not tied to preventable hospitalizations or concentrated among high-risk patients. Health Aff (Millwood). 2017;36(12):2085–93.

32. Zhang H, Cowling DW, Graham JM, Taylor E. Five-year impact of a commercial accountable care organization on health care spending, utilization, and quality of care. Med Care. 2019;57:845–54.

33. NEJM Catalyst. What are bundled payments? 2018. https://catalyst.nejm.org/what-are-bundled-payments/. Accessed 30 July 2019.

34. Barnett ML, Wilcock A, McWilliams JM, et al. Two-year evaluation of mandatory bundled payments for joint replacement. N Engl J Med. 2019;380(3):252–62.

35. Centers for Medicare and Medicaid Services. Bundled payments for care improvement (BPCI) initiative: general information. https://innovation.cms.gov/initiatives/bundled-payments/. Accessed 30 July 2019.

36. Centers for Medicare and Medicaid Services. Bundled payments for care improvement (BPCI) initiative, models 2–4: evaluation years 1 through 3 (through December 31, 2016). https://innovation.cms.gov/Files/reports/bpci2-4-fg-evalyrs1-3.pdf. Accessed 30 July 2019.

37. Centers for Medicare and Medicaid Services. BPCI advanced. https://innovation.cms.gov/initiatives/bpci-advanced. Accessed 30 July 2019.

38. Ballard DJ, da Graca B, Nicewander D, Stauffer BD. Variation in medical practice and implications for quality. In: Nash DB, Joshi MS, Ransom ER, Ransom SB, editors. The healthcare quality book. 4th ed. Chicago: Health Administration Press; 2019. p. 75–106.

39. Fleming NS, Ogola G, Ballard DJ. Implementing a standardized order set for community-acquired pneumonia: impact on mortality and cost. Jt Comm J Qual Patient Saf. 2009;35(8):414–21.

40. Fleming NS, Masica A, McCarthy I. Evaluation of clinical and financial outcomes. In: Ballard DJ, Fleming NS, Allison JT, Convery PB, Luquire R, editors. Achieving STEEEP health care. Boca Raton: CRC Press; 2013. p. 85–92.
41. NEJM Catlyst. What is lean healthcare? 2018. https://catalyst.nejm.org/what-is-lean-health-care/. Accessed 30 July 2019.
42. ASQ Service Quality Division. SIPOC (Suppliers, Inputs, Process, Outputs, Customers) dia-gram. http://asqservicequality.org/glossary/sipoc-suppliers-inputs-process-outputs-customers-diagram/. Accessed 1 Aug 2019.
43. Green RT, Kennerly D. Efficient care. In: Ballard DJ, Fleming NS, Allison JT, Convery PB, Luquire R, editors. Achieving STEEEP health care. Boca Raton: CRC Press; 2013. p. 127–32.
44. Virginia Mason Institute. Who we are. https://www.virginiamasoninstitute.org/who-we-are/#history. Accessed 30 July 2019.
45. Hallam CRA, Contreras C. Lean healthcare: scale, scope and sustainability. Int J Health Care Qual Assur. 2018;31(7):684–96.
46. da Graca B, Filardo G, Nicewander D. Consequences for healthcare quality and research of the exclusion of records from the Death Master File. Circ Cardiovasc Qual Outcomes. 2013;6(1):124–8.
47. Centers for Disease Control and Prevention. Health-related quality of life: surveillance and data. https://www.cdc.gov/hrqol/surveillance.htm. Accessed 30 July 2019.
48. EQ-5D. About EQ-5D. https://euroqol.org/eq-5d-instruments/. Accessed 1 Aug 2019.
49. van Reenan M, Oppe M. EQ-5D-3L user guide: basic information on how to use the EQ-5D-3L instrument. 2015. https://euroqol.org/wp-content/uploads/2016/09/EQ-5D-3L_UserGuide_2015.pdf. Accessed 1 Aug 2019.
50. EuroQoL. EQ-5D-3L. https://euroqol.org/eq-5d-instruments/eq-5d-3l-about/. Accessed 20 Jan 2020.
51. Glick HA, Doshi JA, Sonnad SS, Polsky D. Economic evaluation in clinical trials. 2nd ed. Oxford: Oxford University Press; 2015.
52. McCarthy I, Hostin R, O'Brien M, et al. Cost-effectiveness of surgical treatment for adult spi-nal deformity: a comparison of dollars per quality of life improvement across health domains. Spine Deform. 2013;1(4):293–8.
53. EQ-5D. EQ-5D-3L | FAQs – licensing. https://euroqol.org/eq-5d-instruments/eq-5d-3l-about/faqs/. Accessed 1 Aug 2019.
54. HealthMeasures. PROMIS. http://www.healthmeasures.net/explore-measurement-systems/promis. Accessed 1 Aug 2019.
55. Heath S. Exploring patient reported outcomes measures in healthcare. 2017. https://patien-tengagementhit.com/news/exploring-patient-reported-outcomes-measures-in-healthcare. Accessed 1 Aug 2019.
56. Lavallee DC, Chenok KE, Love RM, et al. Incorporating patient-reported outcomes into health care to engage patients and enhance care. Health Aff (Millwood). 2016;35(4):575–82.
57. HealthMeasures. Intro to PROMIS. http://www.healthmeasures.net/explore-measurement-systems/promis/intro-to-promis. Accessed 1 Aug 2019.
58. Papuga MO, Dasilva C, McIntyre A, Mitten D, Kates S, Baumhauer JF. Large-scale clinical implementation of PROMIS computer adaptive testing with direct incorporation into the elec-tronic medical record. Health Syst (Basingstoke). 2018;7(1):1–12.
59. International Consortium for Health Outcomes Measurement. Standard sets. https://www.ichom.org/standard-sets/. Accessed 22 Jan 2020.
60. Seligman WH, Salt M, la Torre Rosas A, Das-Gupta Z. Unlocking the potential of value-based health care by defining global standard sets of outcome measures that matter to patients with cardiovascular diseases. Eur Heart J Qual Care Clin Outcomes. 2019;5(2):92–5.
61. Imus S. Healthcare cost accounting: 8 strategies to streamline implementation and quickly achieve measurable results. Becker's Hospital CFO Report 2014. https://www.beckershospi-talreview.com/finance/healthcare-cost-accounting-8-strategies-to-streamline-implementation-and-quickly-achieve-measurable-results.html. Accessed 30 July 2019.

62. Ballard DJ, Fleming NS. Rising health care charges: a red herring in a value-based health care world? Mayo Clin Proc. 2019;94(6):946–8.
63. Muir MA, Alessi SA, King JS. Clarifying costs: can increased price transparency reduce healthcare spending? William Mary Policy Rev. 2017;4(2):320–66.
64. Executive order on improving price and quality transparency in American healthcare to put patients first. 2019. https://www.whitehouse.gov/presidential-actions/executive-order-improving-price-quality-transparency-american-healthcare-put-patients-first/. Accessed 30 July 2019.
65. Services CfMaM. Regulation to require drug pricing transparency. Fed Regist. 2019;84:20732–58.
66. National Quality Forum. Measures: cost and efficiency portfolio. http://www.qualityforum.org/Cost_and_Efficiency.aspx. Accessed 30 July 2019.
67. Kaplan RS, Porter ME. How to solve the cost crisis in health care. Harv Bus Rev. 2011;89(9):46–52, 54, 56-61 passim.
68. Porter ME, Pabo EA, Lee TH. Redesigning primary care: a strategic vision to improve value by organizing around patients' needs. Health Aff (Millwood). 2013;32(3):516–25.
69. Social Security Act, 42 U.S.C, §405(r)(1),(5),(6),(8).
70. Social Security Act, 42 U.S.C, §1306c.
71. Agency for Healthcare Research and Quality. All-payer claims databases. https://www.ahrq.gov/professionals/quality-patient-safety/quality-resources/apcd/index.html. Accessed 30 July 2019.
72. Doshi JA, Hendrick FB, Graff JS, Stuart BC. Data, data everywhere, but access remains a big issue for researchers: a review of access policies for publicly-funded patient-level health care data in the United States. EGEMS (Washington, DC). 2016;4(2):1204.
73. Kaiser Family Foundation. Employer health benefits: 2018 summary of findings. http://files.kff.org/attachment/Summary-of-Findings-Employer-Health-Benefits-2018. Accessed 30 July 2019.

Quality Assurance of Data

12

Beverly A. Hardy-Decuir

Introduction

Quality and safe care continues to dominate the interest of the public as well as many health policy agendas. As the leading payer in health care, the Centers for Medicare and Medicaid Services (CMS) defines quality metrics that help health care organizations measure health care processes, outcomes, patient perceptions, and organizational structure and systems. These quality metrics are used by CMS in its quality improvement, public reporting, and pay-for-performance for specific health care providers [1].

This chapter presents a case study that will focus on how a health care organization addressed the quality of data in their quality and safety metrics.

The case study represents a public academic medical center, which will be referred to in the chapter as "the health system." The health system provides primary and specialty care, emergency medicine, and acute hospital care. The mission of the health system encompasses three main objectives: to provide access to quality preventive, acute, and chronic health care regardless of ability to pay; to fulfill the public health needs of the community; and to provide education for patients and health care professionals. While there are many factors contributing to the overall quality of care and services the health system provides to its patients and staff, this chapter will highlight an example of how the health system has embraced improving the quality of the data as an effective strategy for improving quality of care. The strategic plan of the health system reflects the rapidly changing health care environment toward value-based purchasing and other programs that emphasize value over volume as well as greater accountability of health care organizations.

B. A. Hardy-Decuir (✉)
Quality and Clinical Effectiveness, Parkland Health and Hospital System, Dallas, TX, USA
e-mail: beverly.hardy-decuir@phhs.org

© Springer Nature Switzerland AG 2020
P. V. Sreeramoju et al. (eds.), *The Patient and Health Care System: Perspectives on High-Quality Care*, https://doi.org/10.1007/978-3-030-46567-4_12

Case Study

The health system began this initiative in 2015 to accelerate data quality improvement and take a proactive approach by anticipating needs based on upcoming federal and state health policy programs. The changes needed were related to the elements that make up good data: data definitions, data sources, data collection, data validation, data analysis, and data reporting. It was determined that the health system needed a robust data warehouse because some of the data issues were a result of database merges in which the data fields that should be compatible were not due to format inconsistencies.

Background and Approach

Health care data in every health system lives in a complicated web of programs and data systems. Efforts to improve these programs and data systems are frequently delayed due to financial strains with changes in the economy, government budgets, and continually changing health care policies at the federal and state levels [2]. Additional data quality issues identified included:

1. Multiple data system with input from different sources
2. Limited investments in information systems and clinical data analytics
3. Lack of clear definitions for metrics
4. Incorrect encounter data

   The patient data at the health system contains clinical data, health care claims, service patterns of providers, and financial information pertaining to all of these. There is overlapping of financial and clinical data systems and the systems are divided into over 9 subject areas: claim aggregation, financial claims, customers, geography, laboratory, patients, pharmacy, providers, and supplies. There are over 1000 attributes across 4000 columns and over 450 tables. There are many source input files from more than 25 source systems that feed data to the overall data in the health system. Building a data warehouse was already underway in the health system at the time of starting this initiative.

Plan and Rationale

The development of a data quality project plan began with a vision of what quality would mean for the health system. It was developed through discussions with internal and external stakeholders who use data and understand it from a range of perspectives, and with data warehouse team members, who understand past issues, questions, and how they were resolved. The stakeholders included leaders from information systems, financial services, quality management, clinical and nonclinical departments, medical staff, and health information management. The vision provided the basis for a strategy for continual improvement of quality metrics. From this strategy, the health system was able to develop tactics that show results: monitoring of the clinical process of care through clear metrics, reporting on these metrics, recommending and implementing process metrics and process improvements, and demonstrating the impact on the metrics.

The overarching goal was to create a meaningful source of valid, reliable, externally comparable data on how the health system is performing clinically and financially. Ultimately, the project aimed at integrating quality improvement into system processes and providing more reliable data through this integration.

Project Plan

The data quality project plan had four main strategies for implementation [3]. The strategies and tactics are shown in Table 12.1.

The project team listened to the stakeholder's concerns about data, the team's knowledge of data issues, and tracked the issues in a database. End users originally reported many of these issues. The metrics were assessed based on the impact to the database and ownership of data and processes. This allowed for the association of a set of measurable characteristics with each attribute to be monitored. From gathering this information, potential controls were identified and compared with some degree of objectivity. The users learned that the 2015 baseline assessment results showed 77% of the tables met the standard for expected values. They understood that if the patient match did not match the claims, then the processes are not operating as expected. They also know that when an issue is discovered, action is required immediately. Secondly, they know to expect information on a regular basis.

Anticipated impact on subsystems was analyzed in a systematic manner. While the business intelligence team was responsible for maintaining the tables, support

Table 12.1 Implementation strategies and tactics

Strategy	Solution
Obtain management support	Presentation to quality council on current status/practice
	Quarterly status reports
Make approach clear and meaningful	Incorporate approach into processes
	Monthly meetings with stakeholders
	Align incentives
	Develop methods
Build data dictionary	Acquire special software/hardware
	Meetings with data owners
	Meetings with business intelligence
	IT to develop data fields
	Provide all technical assistance
Build credibility with data owners and data users	Monthly data validation
	Submission of error reports to data input owners
	Timely correction of errors
	Perform data conversion before loading into data warehouse

was still needed from other departments to research code definitions. Improving the quality of codes to abstract data depended on support from source system staff that provides definitions for use in the warehouse. Some departments were simply more responsive than others. The process of reviewing tables and researching definitions made clear the role perception played in views on data quality. The metrics differed in importance to end-users. Tables in which few people had a stake were at risk of becoming badly out of date without anyone appearing to notice. In some instances, the data users had other sources for these codes and did not rely on the warehouse version because of which they did not inform the warehouse that updates are needed. The project team identified opportunities for improvement of both the quality of data in the warehouse and through this, of the reputation of the warehouse.

The baseline assessment provided a measure of gross data quality. Through the assessment, the end users were reassured of the quality of data. After the first year, more than 97% of data attributes for VBP met or exceeded the standard. Only eight attributes of 827 did not meet this standard. Several factors contributed to the improved results. A number of one-time issues in the code listings were identified and resolved. With the regular monitoring in place, discrepancies were addressed immediately. For example, automated data quality reports on several of the attributes identified were put in place. This led to improvements in processes associated with these attributes. More efficient assessment processes were implemented. Comparisons between 2015 and 2016 were used to better understand both results and expectations for the data. Because of this, the analysis was more complete and issues and questions were resolved (Table 12.2).

Following on the successful improvement in data quality for metrics included in value-based purchasing, the health system turned to quality measures for specific patient populations. The topics are shown in Table 12.3.

Table 12.2 Summary of improvement in data quality

Data quality domains	Goal	Score	Score before project	Score	Score after project	Score
Completeness	99.0%	1	85.0%	.5	99.0%	1
Acceptable values	99.5%	1	89.5%	.5	99.0%	1
Correct population	99.5%	1	90.0%	.5	95.0%	.5
Timely	99.5%	1	90.0%	.5	92.0%	.5
Resubmissions	5.0%	1	10.0%	.5	5.0%	1
Highest possible data quality score		**5**		**2.5**		**4**

Table 12.3 Future topics for addressing data quality in the health system

Desirable measure	Target population	Condition
Cesarean rate for low-risk first birth women	Children's and maternal health	Perinatal and reproductive health
Adolescent well care visit	Children's health	Utilization
Diabetes short-term complications rate	Chronic disease	Diabetes
Ambulatory care metrics for high-risk populations	Population health	Utilization
Medication treatment for opiate use and alcohol	Adult and adolescent health	Mental health/substance use

Lessons Learned

Implementing the project was a lesson in the relationship between strategy and tactics and what it means to have management buy-in. Both common sense and management theory made it clear that a strategy must be developed before trying to execute tactics. Without a strategy, tactical actions are simply actions; they will lack the coherence and goals needed to move a program forward in a consistent direction. However, this case study shows that successful execution of tactics is also needed for stakeholders to understand project goals and be able to contribute to the strategy. Measuring data quality on an ongoing basis and maintaining the currency of code tables and integrity of keys was helpful for monitoring the impact of changing of one data system on other overlapping data systems. Developing a master data dictionary that contains definitions for all quality metrics and valid code sets and making it available to all stakeholders, including clinical departments was helpful in maintaining credibility and creating reproducibility of the data.

One of the successes of the data quality project was the establishment of metrics that facilitate communication with end users about quality of data in the database. The project created awareness of the importance of aligning the organization's strategic and quality goals with metrics that provide relevant and meaningful information to the patients and the organization.

Conclusion

The data quality project was successful in focusing on improving the quality of data and helped to better manage stakeholder expectations and bridging a previous divide between data owners and data users. The data warehouse became the primary source for a wide range of focused data reports that enabled analysis of health issues, options for care, and delivery of services. The streamlined data reports helped the hospital leadership understand how patients use specific services, how providers treat specific conditions, which treatments are effective, and which care options produce better outcomes. Health care data are complicated, and efforts to streamline them are worthy of the investments required to make them user friendly and meaningful for monitoring quality of care and drive improvements in health systems [4].

References

1. Centers for Medicare and Medicaid Services. Value based purchasing [Fact sheet]. 2017. http://www.cms.gov/medicare/qualityinitiatives.
2. Centers for Medicare and Medicaid Services. Quality measures. 2017. Retrieved from https://www.cms.gov/Medicare/QualityInitiatives-Patient-Assessment-Instruments/QualityMeasures/index.
3. Harris JL, Roussel L, Walters SE, Dearman C. Project planning and management: a guide for CNLs, DNPs, and nurse executives. Sudbury: Jones & Bartlett; 2011.
4. Redman T. Data driven: profiting from your most important business asset. Boston: Harvard Business Review Press; 2008.

Part IV

Humans Caring for Humans

Patient-Centeredness Through Shared Decision-Making

Lynne M. Kirk

In its groundbreaking monograph on improving quality in health care, the National Academy of Medicine (NAM) [1] outlined several characteristics of an optimal health care system for the United States. One of these characteristics is the concept of a patient-centered health care system, focusing health care on the goals and needs of the patient. Central to patient-centered care is the patient's experience of illness and their interactions with the health care system. The Institute for Health Care Improvement [2] incorporated this into its triple aim, along with the outcomes of improved health and affordable cost of care. Patients are often frustrated with their interactions with health care systems, experiencing challenges in participating in decisions about their own health and receiving information in a way that allows them to become informed participants in these decisions.

Patient-Centered Care

Patient-centered care is a health care application that has grown out of a decades-old literature on person-centered care. It was first described by Balint in 1969 [3] as a means to move from practicing "illness-oriented medicine" to practicing "patient-oriented medicine." Patient-centered care has been applied to a variety of personal health services. It is thought to have grown out of Carl Rogers' work in clinical psychology in the 1940s employing client-centered counseling, whereby the clinician creates an environment that allows the client to make the decisions that are right for them [1, 4, 5]. In health care, person-centered care focuses on the biopsychosocial aspects of care and the patient as a person.

L. M. Kirk (✉)
Department of Internal Medicine, UT Southwestern Medical Center, Dallas, TX, USA

Department of Accreditation Services, Accreditation Council for Graduate Medical Education, Chicago, IL, USA
e-mail: Lynne.Kirk@UTSouthwestern.edu

P. V. Sreeramoju et al. (eds.), *The Patient and Health Care System: Perspectives on High-Quality Care*, https://doi.org/10.1007/978-3-030-46567-4_13

Central to patient-centered care is the collaboration between the clinician and the patient for whom they are caring. It also incorporates others involved in the care of the patient including family members and unrelated caregivers. It incorporates the patient's goals, values, preferences, and identified needs. The clinician contributes their own expertise, information about the health condition and possible options and their own values and experiences.

In addition, patient-centered care is provided in a system that focuses on the coordination and integration of care, physical comfort, and emotional support for the patient. There is an intentional component of information, communication, and education of the patient, their friends, family, and caregivers around the patient's health care problems and needs [6].

Patient-centered care has been incorporated into some health care delivery models currently employed. It is very specifically practiced in the patient-centered medical home. This is a model of care that incorporates team-based comprehensive care that is patient-centered, coordinated, accessible, and focused on quality and safety [7]. The patient-centered medical home is usually provided in the primary care setting, but many specialists who treat patients with chronic diseases over long periods of time may also implement this model of care.

Relationship-centered care focuses on the broader range of relationships around the patient, including family members, the community, and the entire team providing patient care [8]. To achieve relationship-centered care, it is important to assure access so that all patients can have a relationship with a health care team to facilitate the patient's care, navigate the health care system, and maintain health. Relationship-centered care also acknowledges the professional relationships among the health care professionals caring for the patient. These facilitate communication and coordination of care.

Shared Decision-Making

An important component of patient-centered and relationship-centered care is shared decision-making in health care [9]. Shared decision-making is the process of jointly making health care decisions based on information exchange between the clinician and the patient to determine the best medical care for the patient in a given clinical situation. It requires that the patient receives accurate and understandable information about the options for assessing or treating their medical problem and that the clinician receives information to understand the patient's goals, values, and preferences and potential barriers to carrying out the agreed upon care. It also importantly requires a shift in the power and control of interactions from the clinician to the patient.

Shared decision-making was originally defined in the early 1980s [10, 11]. It was furthered by discussions regarding the nature of the clinician–patient relationship [12] and informed consent. Shared decision-making goes beyond the clinician providing information to the patient to broad bidirectional information exchange between the clinician and patient to allow the clinical decision to be made that is appropriate for the patient at that time [13]. This type of interaction is termed deliberative by Emanuel and Emanuel.

One criticism of this model is that not all patients want to be as actively involved in their own medical decisions and would rather have the clinician advise them specifically on what to do. There is certainly a range of preferences for medical decision-making based on patient preference and the clinical situation. The information imparted by the clinician, however, remains the same, but at the patient's request, the clinician may provide more guidance on which choice might be made by the patient. Caregivers or family members may also express their perceptions of the patient's wishes about receiving information and participating in decisions. If their perception is that the patient wants less direct involvement, it is important to confirm this directly with the patient prior to withholding information or reducing patient participation in decision-making.

In a review of 115 studies of patients' perceptions of shared decision-making, a majority of patients preferred that method for making their health care decisions. This percentage varied with time of the study with many more preferring shared decision-making in more recent studies. It also varied with the type of illness, with a strong preference for patients diagnosed with serious illness, such as cancer [14].

The strength of the evidence base available for the decision being made will also affect the extent or appropriateness of shared decision-making. If the evidence is strong such that the benefit of the intervention significantly outweighs any risk, the decision may be more clear-cut; however, the patient still needs to be actively involved to make sure that the evidence-based decision is the appropriate one for the patient. If the evidence is not as clear, there may be multiple options with different requirements of the patient and potentially different outcomes, for which the patient's values and preferences are an important component of making the appropriate decision. For example, a patient may have a breast cancer that is amenable to lumpectomy followed by radiation. But because she is located in a rural setting far from a center that can deliver the radiation treatment, she may choose to have a mastectomy and forgo further treatment to avoid the travel and time away from home. The outcome in terms of cancer recurrence may be the same for both treatment options.

In addition to preference-sensitive interventions, shared decision-making may be even more beneficial when the patient has multiple chronic conditions or is older and interactions with other illnesses and time to benefit are more important. Understanding the potential impact of a medical decision on the patient's quality of life may be very important for that patient's decision on whether to undertake such treatment.

The use of shared decision-making has been shown to improve outcomes, especially patients' perceptions of their care. A Cochrane review of studies of shared decision-making using decision aids was published in 2011. In reviewing 86 studies that met review criteria, the investigators concluded that shared decision-making with decision aids improves value-based decision choices, increases patient involvement, and improves knowledge and realistic expectations of outcomes for patients

[15]. An update of that review with six additional years of data again demonstrated increases in patients' perceptions of knowledge, being better informed and clearer about their values. They had a more active role in decision-making and more accurate perceptions of the risk of their health care choices. This review assuredly demonstrated no adverse effects in patient/family satisfaction or health care outcomes [16].

Shared decision-making using decisions aids represents only a subset of care utilizing shared decision-making. Others have looked at the impact of shared decision-making on outcomes of illness in addition to patients' perceptions. In a study of the use of shared decision-making for adults with asthma requiring controller medication, outcomes measured included medication adherence, asthma control, and health care utilization. These were all shown to improve in the patients participating in shared decision-making compared to those receiving usual care [17]. However, a systematic review of thirty-nine studies of shared decision-making (which did not include the asthma study), demonstrated consistent improvements in patients' perceptions of their health care interaction, but failed to demonstrate improvements in health care outcomes in the eight studies where it was measured [18].

Implementing Shared Decision-Making

Once a clinician is convinced that the impact of a shared decision-making on patients is positive, it is important to deliver care in that manner whenever and wherever possible. In addressing this delivery, Elwyn [19] and colleagues have defined and recently refined a three-step model to help overcome some of the barriers for clinicians to engage with patients in shared decision-making. Clinicians frequently perceive barriers as interfering with their ability to employ shared decision-making. These include lack of time, inability to fit it into workflow, and lack of information to provide to the patient for decision-making. The model is designed to overcome these barriers and is built upon providing information to the patient about the decision in a way that they can easily understand the options and the risks and benefits of each. This is followed by supporting the patients in their deliberations in choosing the best option for themselves. This should be done in a way that gives the patient agency in making the decision. The three simplified steps these authors suggest are as follows: (1) team talk; (2) option talk; and (3) decision talk. In the "team talk" step, clinicians outline that they and the patient are working together as a team to describe choices, offer support, and learn about the patient's goals. "Let's work as a team to make a decision that suits you best." At baseline, the clinician determines what the patient already knows about the clinical situation they are in and introduces the plan to discuss the options that are available to address that clinical problem. In the "option talk" step, the clinician discusses all the alternatives with detailed discussion of each option and its risks and benefits to the patient, using risk communication principles outlined below. "Let's compare the possible options."

This may be accompanied by decision support aids if they are available for this clinical decision. The next step, "decision talk," involves making the decision. Eliciting what is important to the patient in terms of outcomes will be helpful to assist in this step. Focusing on how each option might address the patient's goals can help them make the best preference-based decision for them. "Tell me what matters most to you for this decision." If the patient is not ready to make a decision and the next step is not urgent, you can give the patient more time, perhaps along with written materials to help them better understand their options and how those align with their values and preferences. All three talk steps are done using active listening and deliberation.

Implementing these steps is easiest when the clinician and patient are in an ongoing continuity relationship. However, the steps can be implemented in a more acute or consultative setting where the clinician and patient have interacted for a brief period of time or have had no previous interactions.

Meeting the Patient's Needs

Patients must play a central role in shared decision-making. All patients bring expertise to a health care visit. They have the most knowledge of the impact of their symptoms and illness on themselves, their family, and their ability to carry out activities to reach their goals. They also bring the expertise of what they value and what their goals are. They are the most aware of what it will take them to adhere to a plan of treatment and what barriers might exist for that adherence, such as problems accessing food that is necessary to control diabetes and hypertension. Patients also need to be made comfortable enough to share these values, beliefs, and preferences. Probably most importantly they need to be willing to let the clinician know when they do not clearly understand the details of their medical condition or the risks and benefits of the various options for treatment. This ability and willingness to share openly between the clinician and the patient is critical for successful shared decision-making.

Health literacy has been defined as "The degree to which individuals have the capacity to obtain, process, and understand basic health information and services needed to make appropriate health decisions" [1]. A clinical encounter that utilizes shared decision-making requires that the patient receive sometimes complex medical information in a way that they can clearly understand the options. Thus, the patient's health literacy must be considered when presenting this information. Sometimes picture-based tools, such as infographics can be used to more clearly present information to patients regardless of their health literacy. This includes tools or decision aids that spell out absolute risk and benefits and numbers needed to treat or harm. In addition, as our population becomes more diverse, it is important to understand a patient's preferred language and English proficiency. Appropriate use of interpreters is imperative in clinical situations to assure patient understanding.

The Clinician's Role

The health professional serving as the clinician in a health care encounter also has significant responsibilities in undertaking shared decision-making. The clinician needs to explicitly set the stage for the shared decision-making process. This can begin with outlining the decision to be made and the steps required to make that decision and obtaining an agreement to participate in the process from the patient. This may be fairly simple, such as "You've worked very hard on lifestyle changes over the past several months to control your blood pressure. In spite of all that great work, your blood pressure remains above the goal we've discussed for you. I'd like to talk about what the options for further control of your blood pressure are and find which is best for you." If the patient agrees, this can be followed by discussion of the various options and the risks and benefits of each, ultimately leading to the patient and clinician making the decision that the patient and clinician are most comfortable with. If the situation is not urgent, such as the treatment for mildly elevated blood pressure in this example, the patient may want to think it over and defer a final decision until a subsequent communication at a time appropriate for addressing that medical condition.

Estimates of risk must be made on the strongest evidence available from the literature. It is important to communicate risk of various options in a manner that makes it clear to the patient the chances that various decisions may adversely impact him or her. This generally means communicating in terms of absolute risk rather than the relative risk reported in many studies. For example, for a 69-year-old man with treated diabetes and hypertension, deciding on whether to start low-dose aspirin for primary prevention of cardiovascular disease, you would relate that one atherosclerotic cardiovascular disease event is prevented out of seventeen men like him taking daily aspirin over 10 years. Whereas, 1 out of 83 of those men would have a gastrointestinal bleeding episode caused by the aspirin in that 10-year period [20]. An even more clear discussion of this benefit and risk would use a common denominator. Over a 10-year period, out of 100 men taking daily aspirin, 6 would have avoided a heart attack and 1 would have had gastrointestinal bleeding caused by the aspirin [21]. This format is probably helpful for most patients, but especially for those who have limited numeracy.

Incorporating Decision Aids

Sometimes the decisions to be made can be very complex and adequately explaining the risks and benefits of the choices can be a challenge. In this case, decision aids have been helpful in more clearly presenting information to the patient and others who may be helping them with their decision [16]. Decision aids are designed to explicitly portray information related to the risks and benefits of the various options among which the patient and clinician are deciding. A Cochrane review of decision aids outlined the ideal contents of decision aids as follows: (1) provide evidence-based information about the medical condition and the potential benefits, harms, and uncertainties associated with various approaches to the condition; (2)

assist the patient in applying their values to the detailed information about the options available; and (3) guide the steps of the decision and communication about it. Decision aids serve as a complement to the shared decision-making discussion carried out by the clinician and the patient. Such aids may be able to provide additional information for the patient, especially for more complex or high-stake decisions. Most decision aids are paper or electronic communication based, but some may also include videos. The patient (and their caregivers) may want additional time to study the information in the decision aid prior to making a final decision. If possible, the decision can be deferred until the patient and their caregivers can have time to gather all the information they need.

In a clinical area where complex decisions are required repeatedly for certain conditions, it would be worthwhile for the clinical staff to review the decision aids available for those conditions. Those that they feel would be most helpful for their patients can be incorporated into their clinical process and shared decision-making for appropriate patients.

For patients with a shorter life expectancy due to age, serious disease, and/or multiple chronic diseases, shared decision-making incorporating the patient's values and preferences may be even more important [22]. Since most randomized controlled trials that make up the major evidence in clinical decision-making do not include the oldest patients and generally focus on a single illness rather than the multimorbidity present in many elderly patients, clinical decisions for this population may not be as clear-cut as for younger, healthier populations. Consideration of time to benefit and potential for harm becomes even more important. A deeper understanding of the patient's prognosis and goals, values, and preferences are critical for assisting the patient and their caregivers in health care decisions. This includes decisions about treatment and interventions for medical conditions, decisions regarding clinical prevention and screening, and decisions for care in advanced illness. Also important is an understanding of the abilities of the patient and their caregivers to carry out the interventions recommended. This frequently will require consideration of options for community support or a care setting other than the patient's home.

To address these important issues for this population, The American Geriatrics Society has made recommendations for principles to be used in caring for older patients with multimorbidity [22]. These principles incorporate five domains including: (1) patient preferences; (2) interpreting the evidence; (3) prognosis; (4) clinical feasibility; and (5) optimizing therapies and care plan. All of these can be addressed by the teams caring for such a patient within the context of shared decision-making.

Incorporating Shared Decision-Making in Clinical Sites

In your role as a health care professional or a patient, how can you promote the delivery of shared decision-making in the health care setting where you deliver or receive care? The Agency for Health Care Research and Quality has identified several steps to improving care and safety for patients in primary care settings [23].

These steps can be used in multiple health care settings, not exclusively primary care. They provide an effective guide for implementing patient-centered care and shared decision-making in the setting in which you are a clinician. These steps include the following: (1) identify a champion of these efforts in the practice; (2) select the specific strategies to implement to achieve the desired outcome; (3) plan the implementation process; (4) design your implementation; (5) inform patient and family members about the change and encourage them to take part in it; and (6) evaluate the effectiveness of the change in achieving the desired outcomes. For shared decision-making, the steps defined by Elwyn and colleagues and outlined earlier in this chapter may be the processes chosen to implement the change in practice.

If you are a patient or the caregiver or advocate for a patient, you can indicate to the clinicians providing care your preference for patient-centered care and shared decision-making. You can ask them about the choice of clinicians at their health care site who may be able to deliver this care to you. When you see the clinician, you can make sure all of your questions are answered in a way that you fully understand the diagnosis and the choices for care. You can then make sure you effectively communicate to the clinician your goals, values, and preferences regarding this care. These steps should assist you in reaching the appropriate decision for the care you will receive.

Conclusion

This chapter has outlined the genesis of patient-centered care and shared decision-making. The potential benefits of shared decision-making, especially for the experience of care by the patient, have been reviewed. The steps to delivering shared decision-making and incorporating it into a clinical site or practice have been outlined. This information will allow you to go forward as a clinician or a patient to deliver and receive high quality and safe medical care.

References

1. Committee on Quality Health Care in America, Institute of Medicine. Crossing The Quality Chasm: a New Health System for the 21st Century. Washington, D.C.: National Academy Press, 2001.
2. Berwick DM, Nolan TW, Whittington J. The triple aim: care, health, and cost. Health Aff (Millwood). 2008;27(3):759–69.
3. Balint E. The possibilities of patient-centered medicine. J R Coll Gen Pract. 1969;17(82):269–76.
4. Lane L. Client centered practice. Br J Occup Ther. 2000;63(4):310–5.
5. What is person-centered health care? A literature review. (Monograph) National Aging Research Institute. The Victorian Government Department of Human Services, Melbourne, Victoria, Australia, April, 2006.
6. Gerteis ME-LS, Daley J, Delbanco T. Through the Patient's eyes: understanding and promoting patient-centered care. San Francisco: Jossey-Bass Inc.; 1993. 317 p.

7. Defining the PCMH: Agency for Healthcare Research and Quality. Available from: https://pcmh.ahrq.gov/page/defining-pcmh.
8. Chou CL, Hirschmann K, Fortin AH, Lichstein PR. The impact of a faculty learning community on professional and personal development: the facilitator training program of the American Academy on Communication in Healthcare. Acad Med. 2014;89(7):1051–6.
9. Suchman AL. A new theoretical foundation for relationship-centered care. Complex responsive processes of relating. J Gen Intern Med. 2006;21(Suppl 1):S40–4.
10. United States. President's Commission for the Study of Ethical Problems in Medicine and Biomedical and Behavioral Research. Making health care decisions: a report on the ethical and legal implications of informed consent in the patient-practitioner relationship. Washington, DC: President's Commission for the Study of Ethical Problems in Medicine and Biomedical and Behavioral Research: For sale by the Supt. of Docs., U.S. G.P.O.; 1982. p. 1–3.
11. Elwyn G, Frosch D, Thomson R, Joseph-Williams N, Lloyd A, Kinnersley P, et al. Shared decision making: a model for clinical practice. J Gen Intern Med. 2012;27(10):1361–7.
12. Emanuel EJ, Emanuel LL. Four models of the physician-patient relationship. JAMA. 1992;267(16):2221–6.
13. Charles C, Gafni A, Whelan T. Shared decision-making in the medical encounter: what does it mean? (or it takes at least two to tango). Soc Sci Med. 1997;44(5):681–92.
14. Chewning B, Bylund CL, Shah B, Arora NK, Gueguen JA, Makoul G. Patient preferences for shared decisions: a systematic review. Patient Educ Couns. 2012;86(1):9–18.
15. Stacey D, Bennett CL, Barry MJ, Col NF, Eden KB, Holmes-Rovner M, et al. Decision aids for people facing health treatment or screening decisions. Cochrane Database Syst Rev. 2011;(10):CD001431.
16. Stacey D, Legare F, Lewis K, Barry MJ, Bennett CL, Eden KB, et al. Decision aids for people facing health treatment or screening decisions. Cochrane Database Syst Rev. 2017;4:CD001431.
17. Wilson SR, Strub P, Buist AS, Knowles SB, Lavori PW, Lapidus J, et al. Shared treatment decision making improves adherence and outcomes in poorly controlled asthma. Am J Respir Crit Care Med. 2010;181(6):566–77.
18. Shay LA, Lafata JE. Where is the evidence? A systematic review of shared decision making and patient outcomes. Med Decis Mak. 2015;35(1):114–31.
19. Elwyn G, Durand MA, Song J, Aarts J, Barr PJ, Berger Z, et al. A three-talk model for shared decision making: multistage consultation process. BMJ. 2017;359:j4891.
20. Mora, S, Manson, J, Ames, J. Aspirin Guide (Mobile applications software) The Brigham and Women's Hospital, Inc. Boston, MA, 2016. Retrieved from: apps.apple.com/nz/app/aspirin-guide/id1117434628.
21. Edwards A. Risk communication-making evidence part of patient choices. In: Edwards A, Elwyn G, editors. Shared decision-making in health care: Achieving evidence-based patient choice. 2nd ed. Oxford: Oxford University Press; 2009. p. 135–41.
22. American Geriatrics Society Expert Panel on the Care of Older Adults with Multimorbidity. Guiding principles for the care of older adults with multimorbidity: an approach for clinicians: American Geriatrics Society Expert Panel on the Care of Older Adults with Multimorbidity. J Am Geriatr Soc. 2012;60(10):E1–E25.
23. The guide to improving patient safety in primary care settings by engaging patients and families. Rockville: Agency for Healthcare Research and Quality; 2018.

Relationship-Centered Care

14

Krista Hirschmann and Sheira Schlair

Krista's Smile

"Okay, so do you want to do a check-in, or just get down and dirty?" Sheira asked me during our first planning call for this chapter.

The question evoked a broad smile because, for me, that one question encapsulated the goal of this chapter, which is to challenge the widely held belief that there is a tension between task and relationship, when in fact the quality of the relationship determines the quality and efficiency with which the task is accomplished. What might have been a wildly inappropriate question for many other professional situations was simply a short-hand for the years of intense communication training, writing, and co-facilitating that she and I have done together. A check-in would acknowledge that we are each human beings swimming through our respective personal and professional worlds (Sheira a physician-educator, me a social scientist-educator) with competing priorities, distracted thoughts, and corresponding feelings. It would slow us down and help us become more fully present to the work at hand. In contrast, getting "down and dirty" acknowledged that we had rescheduled two planning calls already and had limited protected time prior to our next set of daily responsibilities.

"Just the briefest of check-ins," I responded. "I'm in the car and can't take notes but will be in my destination in 10 minutes."

"I'm at a computer and can take notes," Sheira responded. "How long do you have?" "Fifty minutes at most," I said. "Great," she responded. "I have 45."

K. Hirschmann (✉)
Academy of Communication in Health Care, Allentown, PA, USA

S. Schlair (✉)
Department of Medicine, Montefiore Medical Center, Einstein College of Medicine, Bronx, NY, USA
e-mail: Sschlair@montefiore.org

© Springer Nature Switzerland AG 2020
P. V. Sreeramoju et al. (eds.), *The Patient and Health Care System: Perspectives on High-Quality Care*, https://doi.org/10.1007/978-3-030-46567-4_14

Relationship-Centered Care Everywhere

This anecdote highlights how relationship-centered care recognizes that every technical task without exception takes place in a relational context. The quality of the relationship (and the resultant quality of the communication, trust, and mutual commitment) determines the quality and efficiency of the technical work. Relationship-centered care may sound like another trendy term to confuse and distract from the "real work" of clinical care, but it represents something important for everyone that is worth understanding. Relationship-centered care reflects the shift from thinking about patient care as a one-on-one interaction to patient care as part of a system. Allow us to explain what that means.

In modern times, with the formalization of professional health care training and the increased understanding of clinical science, health care culture has followed a trajectory of elevating the provider (traditionally a physician) from omniscient and benevolent scientist to collaborator and shared decision-maker. This transition has been exemplified in a range of modern portrayals amplified by entertainment, social media, and the content of policy and medical education.

Along this trajectory were two important shifts. The first was in the early 1970s when the term "patient-centered care" entered into circulation in an effort to emphasize that care is about that patient and care needs to be organized around the patient's beliefs, values, agenda, and resources. Patient-centeredness led to an emphasis of new skills sets, such as negotiating with the patient about everything from the goals of treatment to the agenda of an office visit, and continues to remain a central piece of training and healing [1].

Patient-centeredness, however, is an incomplete picture because it focuses solely on the quality of the patient–provider dyad within the clinical encounter. It acknowledges the importance of that particular exchange, but fails to account for the increasing and complex ways for which patients are cared. In her book, *The Antidote to Suffering: How Compassionate Connected Care Can Improve Safety, Quality, and Experience*, Christina Dempsey cites studies "that show that patients may see between 60–100 different caregivers in a single hospital stay," emphasizing that, "Those numbers don't take into account patients' primary care providers, home health nurses, physical therapists, and others who may help with their care both before and after their hospital stay. Patients need to know that all these caregivers are talking to one another," which both reduces waste and, more importantly, prevents harm [2].

The simple point of relationship-centered care is that *both* the connection between the patient and provider *and* the interconnection among the rest of the care team must be strong, as the patient is ultimately cared for and the work accomplished through this network of relationships. (And this tenet is true not just in health care, but in every industry everywhere.) In short, today, it takes many types of relationships to care for a patient and they all count—not just the obvious relationships directly with the patient, but all the backstage, invisible, and indirect ones needed to facilitate care, such as, but not limited to scheduling, pharmacy, administration, housekeeping, food services, security, spiritual and community services, and information technology. As a health care *system*, it takes on the characteristics of any system, meaning ALL of the relationships within it are interconnected (yes, the thought is a little mind boggling.) What's more, health care is influenced by relationships in extended systems, such as education, technology, politics, and related social determinants of health, including leading-edge work to improve housing, nutrition, and employment opportunities to improve health. All of these forces reflect our profound interdependence and how, collectively, any system can potentially enhance or disrupt patient care and provider performance.

To this end, relationship-centered care represents a much more complex perspective that includes increased accountability for personal action and its potential ripple effect. It also, however, recalibrates the values by which clinical care operates [3]. Relationship-centered care is not a transaction, it is an authentic and congruent connection between people in all parts of the system. Ideal? Perhaps. But when we are not valued or treated as human beings, everyone suffers.

Sheira's Phone Call and the Importance of Relationship-Centered Care

I picked up the phone and reflected on the message I needed to share to my long-standing patient, Mrs. Brickman, for whom I served for years as a primary care physician. Proud and stalwart, Mrs. Brickman is an elderly African-American woman with a mistrust of physicians and health care institutions. Mindful of this mistrust, from the early moments of our relationship, I sought to honor her perspectives. Consistent with patient-centered care, we gradually explored and softened this suspicion as we worked together to manage her history of insulin-dependent diabetes. We discussed how her early memories of mistrust originated from as a child growing up in Nashville, Tennessee, pre-Civil Rights movement, and during the era of the Tuskegee Syphilis Study [4]. Over the years, though she remains over her ideal weight, her diabetes has been relatively well controlled and she injects insulin once daily.

Now, I received a message from her insurance company that she would need to transition to a different long-acting insulin as her prior, longtime, long-acting insulin, was no longer going to be paid for by her health insurance company. As I dialed the numbers, I was reminded that, even with mindful and consistent skills, my patient relationships are not immune from the impact of the financial and/or political regulations of health care.

"Mrs. Brickman," I said after we exchanged greetings, "Unfortunately, I have not been successful with getting you the insulin that you've taken for all these years authorized."

Radio-silence. Then in a defensive tone she exclaimed, "Why would you change this on me when I've been so well-controlled? I refuse to change this medication." I felt a 'thud' in my chest. "She doesn't trust me, she's angry with me, I can't fix this unfixable problem, I am so frustrated to work in this system, this is just not fair …" and my mind raced on with automatic negative thoughts as I felt my temperature rapidly rise and tension build in my body. I wanted to say to her "Do you know how frustrated I feel by this entire situation, which I did not create but I have to deal with? This took me time to attempt to get authorization for something that I would not have recommended clinically. I feel tired by the system, I feel drained by this non-clinical administrative work that I'm being asked to do …."

I took a very deep breath while I deliberately engaged in a brief moment of silence. I made the choice to slow down and shifted from information-giver to empathic responder. I then replied, "It sounds like this is coming as a total surprise. I am so sorry to have to break this news to you. And I feel terribly that I was not successful at being able to help you continue your old insulin. I wish it could be different." Another radio-silence. Then she replied with a softer, gentler tone but still with some ambivalence in her tone, and said apologetically "Dr. Schlair, I didn't mean to cross you. This is very upsetting to me, Dr. Schlair. Thanks for trying."

I felt some slight relief in hearing her response, but still felt the weight of my own frustration and exhaustion. I replied as patiently as I could muster, "I am really sorry that I failed to get your old insulin. The person on the other end of the phone explained that you need to try the new insulin and if there is a treatment failure, we can reapply for prior authorization (more administrative work) and are much more likely for it to be approved." I continued, "Mrs. Brickman, you know that I want to help you to the best of my abilities, and I hear your desire to continue with what has really been working all this time. I also wanted to let you know that the other insulin that is now covered by Medicaid may require a bit of a higher dose but is very effective at managing diabetes—pretty much the same as the one you have been on all these years." It was then that I noticed that the tension in my chest had begun to dissipate.

She replied hesitantly "I hear that and I hope it's going to work. I just don't know … I hate when these drugs get changed around. It feels like an experiment—I'm not a lab rat!"

I felt my heart "open," literally felt the tension in my chest dissolve as I took a long breath and replied, "You are not a lab rat. That makes me very sad to imagine what it might feel like to have to say those words. I hope that you never feel that I treat you that way. You are a human being who deserves excellent medical care and to have a chance at controlling your diabetes like you have all these years."

"Yes, Dr. Schlair, I do. Thank you for showing me so much respect," her tone brightened. I felt a swell of emotions and gratitude for her willingness to listen and also to demonstrating her vulnerability.

With the sense that our relationship recalibrated, I moved on to address her "emotional agenda," which often ultimately drives a patient's willingness to engage with their chronic condition and ultimately successfully self-manage their condition(s). "It sounds like you are not comfortable with this situation," I probed. "Do you want to talk more about how it's making you feel or your fears?"

"No Dr. Schlair, I don't want to right now, I'll do my best here with what I've got." "Ok, well you know that I am here, look forward to see you next month, don't forget about our appointment on May 12th."

I ended the call grateful that I had long-standing strong relationship to serve as a safety net. If Mrs. Brickman had been a new patient with the same deep mistrust, I can imagine a much more challenging, perhaps less successful, encounter.

***

Sheira's encounter should come as no surprise to those familiar with the relationship-centered care literature. Indeed, research repeatedly demonstrates that stronger relationships, fostered by skillful communication, lead to a range of desirable outcomes [5]. The Schwartz Center for Compassionate Care summarizes the absence of relationship-centered care on their website: "Unfortunately, the U.S. health care system does not always allow caregivers to establish the kind of strong relationships with patients and families that have been shown to promote health and quality of life. This results in poorer health outcomes, lack of adherence to prevention and treatment recommendations, lower patient satisfaction and higher costs" [6]. Likewise, clinicians feel the direct impact as well. For instance, primary care physicians with more skillful communication experience fewer malpractice suits, and providers supported through interdisciplinary forums designed to "enhance relationships and communication among all members of multidisciplinary health care teams … and to create supportive environments in which all can learn from each other," report increased teamwork and support [7, 8].

The benefits of strengthening relational opportunities within the entire system extend well beyond patients and clinicians, which is particularly important to note, given the immense teamwork necessary to care for patients in both inpatient and outpatient settings.

One framework useful with navigating complexities in relational systems is Jody Hoffer Gittell's framework of Relational Coordination, a theory that pays close attention to the impact of the quality of communication and relationships on the ability of team members to coordinate interdependent tasks, and has generated substantial research specific to health care. This theory has seven dimensions, including frequency, accuracy, and timing of communication, problem-solving communication, shared goals and knowledge, and mutual respect [9].

"Outcomes of relational coordination include efficiency and financial outcomes, quality and safety outcomes, client engagement, worker engagement, as well as learning and innovation" [9]. Relational coordination has also been shown to promote worker satisfaction and resilience, and reduce burnout. In short, when comprised by strong, interconnected relationships, health care has the potential to care not just for the patients who are suffering, but for the millions of health care professionals, both clinical and nonclinical, also suffering due to change fatigue, system inefficiencies, empathic distress, emotional labor, and the countless other issues that drain and dishearten those expected to relentlessly care for others.

Health Care Systems Impact the Homefront

Having finished reading Sheira's story, I leaned back, still staring at the screen, and began thinking how it served as both a poignant and mundane example of the multiple forces challenging a relationship-centered approach, how Sheira not only attended to the patient's concerns, but authentically brought herself to the encounter as well by naming her motives and apologizing for the limitations of her influence. I thought about the people involved with changing the Medicaid formulary, the processes, and relationships in their system and behind their decisions, and if they ever imagined the myriad of ways these small changes potentially impact clinical relationships and sometimes impede care.

"Did I tell you the story about Walmart?" my husband, a family physician, asked, interrupting my thoughts.

"No," I responded half-listening and a little annoyed with the distraction.

"Their pharmacy wants us to send them patient records for any prescription of a controlled substance."

"All of their records?" I clarified, processing the implications.

"Yea, and if I was a patient, I'd be livid to find out that my records were leaving the office. Pharmacies started doing this a couple of years ago because Medicaid required them to ask for office notes for diabetic patients, but sometimes there's other things not related to diabetes in the note that they don't need to see. It's just one more thing that can erode trust and ding physician autonomy," he said, temporarily concluding his venting.

"So I hear," I acknowledged looking at his weary face and then glancing back to the screen. "That sounds frustrating to have yet one more task put upon what I know is very full plate for a busy office," I said, having learned over the years when to offer an analytical comment, and when to simply to reflect and empathize over an imperfect system.

***

It's easy, writing from the frontline perspective, to point fingers at the faceless hands of power and influence—insurance companies, politicians, administrators, supply chains, IT companies— whose ability to change the coverage, the laws, the policies, the equipment, and the technology creates a sea of constant and exhausting change. And yet (much to our own dismay sometimes), systems thinking, and by extension, relationship-centered care does not accommodate scapegoating. Blaming one part of the system is antithetical to the idea that it is what happens *between* the parts, not the parts themselves that create the outcomes. To reference the often-quoted Paul Batalden, "Every system is perfectly designed to get the results that it gets" [10].

Sheira Experiences Relationship-Centered Care in Action

It was a Saturday morning clinic half-day. I walked into the room of my first patient, Mr. Gerhart, for whom I had been a primary care physician for just a few months after he transferred from his previous long-standing provider after they had recently left the clinic. The patient had a distant history of alcohol dependence (now in remission) and had been prescribed alprazolam ("Xanax") for several years for an unclear indication and was taking it multiple times daily when I met him. I had reluctantly continued the prescription and had decided, along with the guidance of my medical director and clinic psychiatrist, that this was not a safe long-term treatment for what I had determined was likely generalized anxiety disorder. The team had decided that he would need to seek psychiatric consultation to help clarify his psychiatric diagnosis and treatment, and that it was no longer appropriate for him to receive alprazolam from primary care.

He had shared with me over the past several visits that he felt that the alprazolam was cutting cravings and improving his sleep. He had declined referral to a psychiatrist for assessment, and a recommendation to go back to Alcoholics Anonymous for ongoing peer support, both of which I believed would be useful means to manage his cravings, anxiety, and insomnia.

Before I entered the room, I considered both my message and approach in sharing that I could no longer safely fill the alprazolam, and that I would refer him expeditiously to a psychiatrist for consultation. I felt fear rise in my chest as pressure increased from my racing heart. I worried, "This is going to be potentially messy, and he might get very angry." I closed my eyes and repeated a few times under my breath "Tread lightly. Slow down." When I walked in the room, sat down, and opened my stance at a half angle, making eye contact with Mr. Gerhart. I smiled and began a social question by asking, "How is your wife doing?" After a short exchange, I asked him for his goals for the visit today and he replied, "I need my Xanax refilled, that's about it." I told him "Well that's my agenda item today too, so we can focus on that. What else?" He said, "That's all I have to discuss, no medications need refilling otherwise, and no other issues."

I then acknowledged, "So I know how much you feel that Xanax has been helping you all these years and that you feel that you need to continue it. I wanted to let you know that along with our team, we are concerned that the Xanax is not a safe medication to take long term. We recommend that you see a psychiatrist to assess how to handle your feelings of anxiety."

He said gruffly and with an anxious and angry lilt, "I'm not seeing a shrink…. What's the big deal? It's helped me all this time, I'm not drinking, and that's a win!" I felt fear in my chest, took a breath and responded, "Well, I cannot safely refill the Xanax. I see it as a win that you have not been drinking all this time, and recognize that you feel cravings to drink when you feel anxious, and that Xanax calms your nerves. I get that. We need an expert view to weigh in on how we can more safely manage your anxious feelings long term." His stance was visibly closed, arms crossed.

"Mr. Gerhart, remember how we talked about the potential for short-acting medications like Xanax (or alcohol) to cause your body to become dependent on the medication?" He nodded with his eyes looking downwards and his arms still crossed "Yeah."

"Well, I believe that not only is your body now showing signs of dependence on Xanax so that when you don't get it, you go through withdrawal. In fact, your anxiety is likely at least partially if not all because your body is withdrawing from the Xanax. But also, we need to know what we are treating!" There are lots of different kinds of anxiety that needs all different sorts of treatments. I'm not the safe expert to do this. A psychiatrist is."

He was stone cold silent, now looking increasingly more agitated. I felt numb.

"Mr. Gerhart, are you willing to see a psychiatrist? That is the only way that we can go. I will refill your Xanax until that appointment and we will make you an appointment on Monday when the social worker comes back and call you with a psychiatric appointment as soon as possible."

He suddenly stood up, wrung his hands and his vocal tone immediately escalated. He yelled "F- you, Dr. Schlair, you [expletive]. I will use whatever I need, it's because of you that I am going to have to go back to drinking …"

I felt physically threatened, felt my pulse suddenly racing, and I stood up and moved toward the door and while holding the door handle said, "Do not raise your voice at me." And then, I exited the room. I took several minutes to breath, I spoke with a nurse about what had just happened. We decided that we would go back in the room and ask him to please depart the clinic. When I returned, he was still visibly angry and he left without incident.

The next week, the clinic administration and I met to discuss what had happened on my request and it was suggested that he and I discuss termination and/or transfer of care to a different physician. An appointment was made soon thereafter and at our next appointment, we were both calm and spoke respectfully, he expressed his shame and frustration and apologized for how he had spoken to me. I expressed my continued concern for his well-being and belief that he would be best served by a new provider given the line that had been crossed, which to me felt like a breakdown of trust. He agreed and expressed understanding about that. He also expressed appreciation for the relationship that we had had and I expressed agreement with that. He agreed to see another provider and that he would consider a psychiatric consultation and voiced understanding that the alprazolam was not a safe long-term option. During the appointment, I expressed my appreciation for his apology and respect for his emotions and needs, and gratitude for having been his doctor. He shared his gratitude for our relationship and desire that things could have been different, and feeling of shame that he had 'crossed that line.'

While this might be an extreme example and not representative of the average physician–patient encounter, our ongoing communication epitomizes the essence of relationship-centered care, particularly with my consistent effort to express PEARLS during each interaction (Partnership, Empathy, Apology, Respect, Legitimation, Support) [5]. While in extreme cases relationship management may be the domain of behavioral specialists, we forget that doctors are humans too and that even the most experienced and compassionate doctors are challenged by some patient relationships. There is the caring aspect and there is the responsibility aspect. Learning how to successfully navigate a healthy boundary between the two is an ongoing lesson.

Meanwhile, at the time of this critical incident and thereafter, I had been caring for his wife as well, for whom he is the primary caregiver. At her next visit and over subsequent years, we have maintained a very warm and cordial relationship in all of her appointments, to which he consistently accompanied her. The power of relationship-centered communication is demonstrated in how our relationship has survived this critical incident intact, to the extent that she passed away this year unexpectedly and tragically, and he invited me to her funeral, accepted my condolences, and warmly expressed appreciation for my care of her and of him.

Achieving Relationship-Centered Care Together

Taking a break from a morning of research at home, I (Krista) reluctantly wandered into my children's bathroom, and began scrubbing the dried toothpaste out of their sink. Flipping on a Freakonomics Radio podcast for company, I randomly selected an episode titled, "The Most Ambitious Thing Humans Have Ever Attempted" (April 25, 2018). Lured by the grandiose promise as a distraction from my task, I imagined learning about space travel to Mars, or constructing the tallest building in the world. But, alas, no. It turns out that "The Most Ambitious Thing Ever" is fixing the high spend and low quality of US health care. Sigh. The invited guest was surgeon and author, Atul Gawande and as he and Steven Dubner bantered in the background, a particular comment caught my attention. Dr. Gawande explained:

There's a fundamental disconnect often between the academic work and the work needed to answer the key questions that people in the political sphere are trying to answer. Often people are trying to come to experts for technical answers to questions that don't have a technical answer … The case in point is the Affordable Care Act. The trouble is that people fundamentally disagree on what the goal of the health coverage is. Is it to free up a trillion dollars for a tax reform? Is it to secure universal coverage for all? Is it to cut costs? You can't take a trillion dollars out of the health care system and make health care better at the same time and increase coverage in a short timeframe [11].

The trouble is that people fundamentally disagree on what the goal is. And suddenly I was transported to my former role of coaching primary care offices where we might ask, "What is the goal of where the patient should be at 9:00 for a 9:00 appointment? (a) walking in the door (b) finished checking-in (c) being roomed (d) speaking with the provider. It was not unusual to get 3–4 different answers even in a small office!

These conversations were then guided by the framework of relational coordination, mentioned above, as a way to measure the strength of tie, or interdependence, within a relational system. Although seven different dimensions guide the framework, we always started with conversations about goals. What are we trying to achieve together? If we don't start with shared goals, then the rest of the work is incredibly complicated, frustrating, and difficult because we are chasing different outcomes.

So what is the goal of a relationship-centered care?

The simple answer is that because the work gets done through the relationship, the goal is to always act in a way that, at minimum, seeks to preserve the relationship and, at best, seeks to strengthen it.

As relational coordination would remind us, however, it is not enough to share a goal. From a systems perspective, we must also understand *one another's responsibilities* (not just our own) with accomplishing the work needed to achieve that goal. Any part of any system, including relational systems, inherently impacts the other parts either by design or by accident. While we can never fully anticipate these impacts, we can create regular opportunities to deliberately recognize our interdependence on others and have conversations that ask questions like, "How does the way I do my work affect your ability to do yours?" (Suchman, A, personal communication 2016)

With both the goal of relationship-centered care defined, and the mutually influential role we each play acknowledged, how can relationship-centered care facilitate its own propagation? Admittedly, it would be easy to turn to lofty platitudes that would provide ambiguous direction and mild inspiration, but we don't think that it is fair to shield you from specific answers just because they require real work.

Relationship-centeredness, including patient care, clinical education, administration, and interprofessional teamwork, requires multiple levels of investment beginning with the following:

1. Developing Personal Awareness: Personal awareness is the foundation for all other levels of investment. There are many avenues and resources available to explore this territory and support attempts to recognize blind spots, identify strengths, categorize personality type, uncover our unconscious biases, check assumptions, and reflect on major life influencers, such as our families of origin. Undoubtedly, personal awareness can be a challenging and emotional journey. Having a trusted source for feedback and reflection while you stretch toward new perspectives can be immensely helpful.

2. Patient and Caregiver Activation: Patients and caregivers may also need to reconceptualize their roles. They need to be active participants, prepare for visits with talking points and questions, and even be ready to point out when they feel that the clinician has not understood them and expressing appreciation when they have. Patients and caregivers can also enhance their empowerment and effective communication through variety of resources, including the Institute for Patient and Family Centered Care [12].

3. Communication Skills Training: While communication skills training and simulation patients are increasingly popular in clinical education programs, and we applaud these efforts, often, we find they are not enough, particularly once the strain of regular clinical practice has taken its toll. As with anything, it is easy to develop sloppy habits and unhealthy routines that might feel comfortable, but are ultimately undermining good intentions. For example, the Academy of Communication in Health Care, an interprofessional home to health care professionals who have an interest in promoting relationship-centered care, offers specialized communication training to refresh and improve upon basic skills for health care providers [13].

4. Facilitated Conversations of Interdependence: As this entire chapter has laid out, it is not enough to effectively communicate with just the patient. Rather, team members must utilize these same basic communication skills and make concerted efforts to seek feedback from one another. Regularly asking for feedback from co-workers in a safe and well-facilitated environment minimizes implicit power differentials and makes transparent the coordination required to accomplish goals.

5. Congruent Leadership: Finally, the first four levels of investment must be supported by congruent leaders who recognize the centrality of relationships in the workplace, who seek to develop themselves as authentic and congruent human beings, including permission to express vulnerability, and who, as a result, lead from a socio-technical perspective rather than purely relying on technical strategies and approaches [14, 15].

Together, these five levels of investment are a starting place for seeding relationship-centeredness. No one approach is enough, however, and, ultimately, they must be married to creative organizational structures and proven technological approaches as well to support and sustain a dynamic relational system [14, 15]. Make no mistake though, starting with the technical side is like trying to build a house without first pouring a foundation. The structure might look wonderful, but the slightest storm will lead to instability and collapse. In organizations, this manifests as a fear-based culture that amplifies the challenges of embracing interdependence and optimally coordinating work.

Call to Action

We have referenced a number of specific resources in this chapter that foster relationship-centered care, toward which we are openly and unapologetically biased. Our bias stems from witnessing thousands of health care professionals and patients benefiting from adoption of these skills and resources over the past two decades. And, we can assure you that cultivating the necessary skills to recognize internal tensions and deliberately attend to them in the moment is not easy or quick. The alternative, however, produces a greater cost, literally, than investing in approaches that support and strengthen relational systems. These investments result in better outcomes for both the work itself and the people performing it. The call to action is to prioritize relationships first and foremost, beginning with ourselves and our local systems.

Epilogue

Krista: Well, we hit our 5000 words. How do you hope and think it will land on readers?

Sheira: I hope that what we wrote about resonates with them and even touches them. I would hope that they would have a deeper appreciation for the challenge and the gift of slowing down.

Krista: Yes, and I also hope that they realize that slowing down relationally, embracing differences, and connecting authentically may actually help to accelerate identifying and meeting the goals that we're trying to achieve in health care.

Sheira: I would want a reader to walk away with a deeper appreciation for the role that we all play in a system. And to think to herself when she goes to the doctor's office the next time, that the system is often complex and frustrating for health care professionals too. Odds are that the clinicians are likely trying their best to be an effective advocate.

Krista: And … it would be wonderful if some readers could commit to enhancing their own personal awareness, communication skills, or perhaps invite feedback as a team member or a leader. We are inherently interdependent, and therefore we are each accountable to building, repairing, sustaining relationships through effective communication practices. Only through such efforts can we create an optimal health system while mindfully relating to one another as human beings.

References

1. Beach MC, Inu T, Relationship-Centered Care Research Network. Relationship-centered care: A constructive reframing. J Gen Intern Med. 2006;21:S3–8.
2. Dempsey C. The antidote to suffering: how compassionate connected care can improve safety, quality, and experience. New York: McGraw-Hill; 2018. p. 93.
3. Kohn LT, Corrigan JM, Donaldson MS. To err is human: building as safer health system. Washington, DC: The National Academic Press; 2000.
4. The notorious Tuskegee Syphilis Study began in 1932 as a joint effort between the Public Health Service and the Tuskegee Institute in order to track the natural progression of syphilis in 600 black men, 399 of whom were infected. Lasting for 40 years instead of the intended six months, the study was later declared "ethically unjustified" for failing to provide treatment even once penicillin became widely known and available as an effective drug. (https://www.cdc.gov/tuskegee/timeline.htm). Most importantly, "It destroyed the trust many African Americans held for medical institutions—a legacy that persists today." (https://www.washingtonpost.com/news/retropolis/wp/2017/05/16/youve-got-bad-blood-the-horror-of-the-tuskegee-syphilis-experiment/).
5. Chou C, Cooley L, editors. Communication RX. New York: McGraw-Hill; 2018.
6. https://www.theschwartzcenter.org/redefining-quality-care/national-consensus-project/.
7. Levinson W, Roter DL, Mulloly JP, Dull VT, Frankel RM. The relationship with malpractice claims among primary care physicians and surgeons. JAMA. 1997;277(7):553–9.
8. Lown BA, Manning CF. The Schwartz Center Rounds: evaluation of an interdisciplinary approach to enhancing patient-centered communication, teamwork, and provider support. Acad Med. 2010;85(6):1073–81.
9. Hoffer Gittell J. New directions for relational coordination theory. p. 400. https://rcrconnect.org/resource-center/outcomes-and-predictors/.
10. http://www.ihi.org/communities/blogs/origin-of-every-system-is-perfectly-designed-quote.
11. Freakonomics Radio. The most ambitious thing humans have ever attempted. April 25 2018. (13:00). https://www.wnycstudios.org/story/most-ambitious-thing-humans-have-ever-attempted/.
12. http://www.ipfcc.org/.
13. https://www.achonline.org/.
14. Hoffer Gittell J. Transforming relationships for high performance: the power of relational coordination. Stanford: Stanford University Press; 2016.
15. Suchman A, Sluyter DJ, Williamson PR. Leading change in healthcare: transforming organizations using complexity, positive psychology, and relationship-centered care. London: Radcliffe Publishing; 2011.

When Technical Solutions Are Not Enough: Engaging Everyone in Improving Health Care

15

Lucía Durá

> Relationships exist between things. You can point at things, but you can't point at relation-ships. They are literally hard to see. – Frances Westley, Brenda Zimmerman, and Michael Patton in *Getting to Maybe* ([1], p. 10)

I remember sitting in a reclining chair in a podiatrist's office cringing as he worked to extract an ingrown toenail. Thanks to the local anesthetic, I couldn't feel any-thing, but I had to work hard to keep myself distracted. The best thing that came to mind was to look through a magazine while singing in my head. In the middle of the procedure, the doctor looked up at me and said, "I need a nurse. Hang on."

Without getting up from his rolling stool, the doctor glided to the door, and I watched as he put one gloved hand on the door handle and another on the door-frame, peeking outside and calling the nurse's name. The nurse said she'd be right over, and he rolled back to work on my toe.

He smiled and said, "Ready?"

"Yes," I assented.

But I wasn't ready. Familiar with proper hand hygiene procedures, I wanted him to remove the gloves, wash his hands, and put on new gloves. Instead, he simply picked up where he left off. And I cringed even more than before, heart racing, wishing to disappear, hoping that the ordeal would end quickly, painlessly, and ulti-mately without infection.

On the drive home, I replayed the situation in my head. I should have said no when the doctor asked if I was ready for him to go back to the procedure. I said nothing. I was scared, but of what? I'm a PhD who studies health communication, *specifically* infection prevention and patient safety protocols. Still, on the day I was the patient, I let a doctor treat an open wound with the same gloves that had just

L. Durá (✉)

Department of English, The University of Texas at El Paso, El Paso, TX, USA

e-mail: ldura@utep.edu

© Springer Nature Switzerland AG 2020

P. V. Sreeramoju et al. (eds.), *The Patient and Health Care System: Perspectives on High-Quality Care*, https://doi.org/10.1007/978-3-030-46567-4_15

touched the door handle and the doorframe. I resented myself for not speaking up, and I resented him for not being my advocate after placing my trust in him. Fortunately, my toe healed without infection. But every time I made a payment toward my balance on the procedure, I felt a pang of regret. My experience with the podiatrist helped me confirm two things first-hand. First, patient safety doesn't discriminate on the basis of situational or demographic characteristics—even a so-called "educated" person is vulnerable as a patient and can use an advocate. Second, patient safety is as much a matter of communication as it is about protocols and policies.

Inspired by the need to examine and improve the less visible and relational aspects of health care, in this chapter, I explore the assumptions of hierarchical thinking and complexity thinking and how these affect the ways we communicate and solve health care problems. I discuss two frameworks that can help us engage *everyone* in finding solutions to difficult problems: Discovery and Action Dialogues and Improv Prototyping. These frameworks have been applied in health care, usually as part of Positive Deviance interventions, which focus on identifying small, local solutions making a difference in addressing big, intractable issues, e.g., infection prevention and patient safety (see [2] and [3], p. 86). Discovery and Action Dialogues offer an inquiry framework to ask what are some of the things that individuals, including patients, their families, doctors, nurses, and other less usual contributors like volunteers and clergy, are already doing to solve a problem, e.g., prevent health care-associated infection (HAI) spread? As a complementary or stand-alone action-based framework, Improv Prototyping helps us deepen our understanding of successful practices by unearthing the tacit, creative, step-by-step behaviors and communication patterns that help individuals work around named challenges. I end the chapter with concluding thoughts around communication and courage.

Not Just People but the Spaces Between People

Patient safety encompasses quite a bit, from errors and injuries to accidents and infections. In this chapter, I focus on HAI because it is the area of patient safety with which I have the most experience as a communication consultant. HAI are preventable, and they are very clearly on the radar of national, state, and local health care organizations. Walk into any health care facility in the USA and you will notice countless HAI prevention signs aimed at clinicians, cleaning staff, patients, and visitors. Indeed, organizations like the Centers for Disease Control and Prevention (CDC) and the Association of State and Territorial Health Officials (see [4]) fund toolkits for facilities to use. If health care facilities train staff and post, distribute, and maintain signage and reminders, why do HAI continue to be so prevalent? In my experiences doing research at hospitals, clinicians often point the finger at patients and visitors. And certainly, raising awareness across the board is important. Yet, no matter who we are among the stakeholders, what we lack, I argue, is not *just* awareness of HAI transmission and protocols. We lack (1) reflexivity about our own role(s) in prevention and/or (2) how that role is connected to others' roles, i.e., how it functions in a social web.

In general, communication within health care organizations follows a hierarchical model. Stakeholders work together in very specific ways, with clear roles: doctor–patient, nurse–doctor, administrator–custodian, etc. Such relational structures serve the system well in facilitating things like order, process, and replication. Further, these role structures are compatible with evidence-based practices, which in addition to privileging the scientific method and knowledge from randomized controlled trials [5] are growing to consider clinician experiences and patient values [6]. Even so, the evidence-based practice model focuses on a very small social web: patient, clinician, and data. Undergirding this model are two important assumptions about the "vast majority" of people operating within the health care system, i.e., every single person who walks through a health care facility door: patients, caregivers, family members, custodial staff, food services staff, maintenance staff, volunteers, clergy, etc. These assumptions are that "the vast majority":

1. Have little or nothing to contribute that could make a significant difference (i.e., [sic] bottom-up is useless)
2. Will be willing (i.e., [sic] will offer no resistance) and capable of rapidly and effectively implementing decisions from which it was excluded [7]

In essence, the vast majority are simply supposed to follow the signs, protocols, and orders to which they have access. But that's not quite working, is it? What if we included the vast majority in not only complying with but also *designing and implementing* patient safety initiatives, such as infection prevention campaigns? What I am proposing here is that while the vast majority's local, context-driven behaviors may not "count" as evidence-based practices, they can be accounted for as *practice-based evidence* [8, 9]. Practice-based evidence includes the local, context-driven behaviors of *all* participants within a health care facility that contribute to mitigating patient safety issues. Practice-based evidence can help elucidate how roles are interconnected, and it can be produced by engaging everyone.

Engaging everyone requires that we suspend our assumptions about the vast majority, and in doing so, that we also suspend our assumptions about experts. This does not mean we throw out evidence-based practices or hierarchical roles out of the windows. It means paying attention to how communication is networked. We can do this by taking a page from complexity theory. In contrast with the assumptions of hierarchical thinking, two assumptions of complexity thinking are that

1. The vast majority is capable of complex, collective problem-solving that adapts to changing situations.
2. Just as valuable as the nodes in a network is what is happening in between them, i.e., the spaces between people.

Complexity in health care is not new. Scholars and practitioners have described health care systems as complex for years [10–14]. To explain the differences among simple, complicated, and complex, Westley, Zimmerman and Patton [1] use the examples of baking a cake (as simple), sending a rocket to the moon (as complicated), and raising a child (as complex). In simple and complicated situations, protocols and replication are both possible and valuable. Because of this, there is a high degree of certainty in outcomes. In complex situations, protocols and replication do not guarantee the same outcomes.

Health care systems encompass simple and complicated aspects, but the fact that they (health care systems) can't be reduced to any one aspect and that they exist in a social milieu, makes them complex. Despite the general awareness of complexity in health care, we are quick to execute and latch onto simple and complicated solutions because of our evidence-based mentality. As Glouberman and Zimmerman [10] explain, we think that statistical correlations "will provide a causal deterministic account of health with a high degree of predictability. This is not really the case. There is often little proof of the direction of the causality, uncertainties are ignored and the resulting pictures tend to ignore the picture of health as complex, probabilistic, with many factors interacting not only with the individual but also with each other" (p. 11). Glouberman and Zimmerman [10] provide a detailed account of the differences between complicated and complex thinking/approaches to various areas such as disease, theory, evidence, causality, evidence, and planning. These differences are worth considering so that we don't treat things like raising a child like baking a cake, or even like sending a rocket to the moon. Westley, Zimmerman, and Patton [1] cite the example of mental health solutions that focus on "engineering the correct psycho-pharmaceutical intervention" (p. 10). Such solutions are evidence based and can be both efficient and effective, but they ignore that patients are often (1) too ill to adhere to prescribed drug regimens, and (2) in need of support systems that respond to their needs and circumstances. In other words, patients are embedded in relational webs, which are rarely factored into care, particularly when the evidence-based factor has been checked off and decisions are pressured by urgency, efficiency, and economic sense.

Let me reiterate that linear approaches, technical solutions, and well-functioning protocols are not in opposition to complexity. The goal is to complement these with complex-based approaches. And while it may seem that urgency, efficiency, and economic sense are jeopardized by the time investment in human capital, investing in social, relational aspects has actually been shown to improve patient safety and overall stakeholder engagement [15]. In the section that follows, I describe two frameworks used in a Positive Deviance intervention that emphasize the value of practice-based evidence, the spaces between people, and interconnectedness.

Positive Deviance: Engaging Everyone in Practice-Based Evidence

In 2008, the *New York Times Magazine* featured an article as part of its 8th annual Year in Ideas issue on Positive Deviance, or PD. PD assumes that in every community where there is an intractable problem, there are people who have already found solutions without outside help. The key is in finding these individuals or groups and identifying their successful practices so that they can be adopted by the larger community.

This article covered how PD was being used to address HAI in US hospitals by focusing on the solutions—not the problem—and by engaging everyone. It cited two examples that have become cornerstones in conversations about complexity and HAI. The first example described contributions to HAI prevention at the VA hospital in Pittsburgh from custodial staff and clergy: room cleaning checklists and Bible slipcovers. These small behaviors, which came from the least expected places, i.e., non-clinical individuals, contributed to a 50% decrease in infections at the Pittsburgh VA hospital [16, 17].

The second example, drawn from HAI prevention work using PD at Albert Einstein Medical Center in Philadelphia, even has its own YouTube video showing what is now known in complexity circles as the "Palmer Method." The Palmer Method was a technique that Jasper Palmer, a transport worker, developed to take off his gown upon exiting a patient's room in a way that rolled it to minimize contamination and that also ended up compressing it, which facilitated disposal while decreasing trash volume.

The PD approach is grounded in complexity and values inclusion and small, everyday practices, which are generally overlooked in more traditional problem solving, as sustainable sources of innovation. What is perhaps less obvious about these examples of PD in health care is that they did not exist in a vacuum. Engaging everyone at Albert Einstein led to a drop in infections; it also led to culture change. People started to communicate more respectfully, share stories, and suggest ideas or improvements [18]. In the words of a hospital employee, Maureen Jordan, "I was used to identifying a problem and getting the correction implemented, 1,2,3....Now it's not just me preaching. It's people feeling they have created something that they own" (quoted in [18], p. 90). In essence, PD generated a momentum toward culture change because it engaged everyone and foregrounded the practice-based evidence that was making a difference.

Embedded in PD are dynamic inquiry and conversation frameworks that facilitate trust building, information gathering, and grassroots implementation. Two of these frameworks have become tried and true in PD projects dealing with patient safety, specifically HAI prevention: Discovery and Action Dialogues and Improv Prototyping. Both of these frameworks are grounded in complexity theory and have been systematized by practitioners, forming part of the menu of Liberating Structures, or LS [19]. LS are alternatives to conventional structures, e.g., presentations, managed discussions, status reports, brainstorms, and open discussions. Licensed under Creative Commons, anyone can use them. LS aim to help people work with groups more effectively by offering ways to include, engage, and promote creativity and ownership among stakeholders.

I had the opportunity to participate in the design and facilitation of Discovery and Action Dialogues (DAD) at a public academic hospital in Dallas. This work was part of a study funded by the University of Texas System Patient Safety to evaluate whether the implementation of PD in a group of three hospital wards decreased HAI incidence, in contrast to a control group of three wards that did not receive PD intervention. The DADs were implemented by two local team members, including the project lead, over a period of 5 months—I would fly in once a month. In those 5 months, the team conducted a total of 54 DADs with 110 participants. We would conduct them in the way that was most convenient to the staff in the three wards, e.g., one-on-one conversations, focus groups, anonymous drop box, and graffiti board reporting in break rooms. And we included patients, families, and other hospital staff as much as possible.

According to the Liberating Structures' DAD description, "DADs make it easy for a group or community to discover practices and behaviors that enable some individuals (without access to special resources and facing the same constraints) to find better solutions than their peers to common problems" [20]. DADs in health care tend to be carried out in local units in groups, standing or sitting, and can take anywhere from 15 minutes to more than an hour—whatever the context allows. We adapted the framework to our setting and used the following protocol [21]:

1. How do you know or recognize when HAI is present?
2. How do you protect yourself, patients, and others from transmission of any microorganisms?
3. What prevents you from taking these actions all the time?
4. Is there any group or anyone you know who is able to overcome the barriers frequently and effortlessly? How?
5. Do you have any ideas?
6. What initial steps need to be pursued to make it happen? Any volunteers?
7. Who else needs to be involved?

DADs' value in health care is derived from the fact that, although there seem to be protocols for everything in clinical practice, several bedside practices don't have protocols, or the order of the steps within each protocol is not clear, which leaves clinicians to fill in the blanks and come up with their own ways. These "innovations" are rarely communicated, often because they become embedded in everyday practice. But harvesting and nurturing these ideas is a low-cost quality and culture improvement opportunity.

The 54 DADs yielded 210 ideas. The ideas were vetted by the health care epidemiology team for actual infection prevention effectiveness and by the study team for replicability and innovativeness. These were the top 10 ideas that merged practice and evidence:

- Asking dietitian to wash hands between patient visits. Dietitian now calls patients when s/he can to avoid going into the room.
- Removing urinals and bedpans from the side table.
- Remind each other to reinforce use of PPE.
- Do one-glove method, which is using one-gloved hand to handle chemotherapy waste or food trays in the isolation room, and the ungloved hand to turn the doorknob.
- If patients have infectious pathogens, give them informational handout.
- Order test for *Clostridioides difficile* when patient admitted with diarrhea or develops diarrhea.
- Pump hand sanitizer dispenser twice when entering the room, while interacting with patient, and when leaving room (total six times when I see patient).

- Have patients (and families) change into a new gown if in contact isolation and leaving room.
- Educate families to keep objects in room if patient is in contact isolation, and other precautions.
- Tell family to wash their hands and to remind staff to wash hands and wear a gown if they fail to do so.

Some of these ideas required further exploration or expansion to get to the more concrete, replicable behaviors behind them. For example, when you say educate the families, how do you do this? What if there are language barriers? What if you have different family or visitors all the time? This is where we decided to employ Improv Prototyping.

We facilitated six Improv Prototyping sessions, calling them more informally, "What if" role-playing sessions since we found "What if" to be a useful scenario structure. Different from the DAD interviews in which we adapted to specific staff schedules in each ward, we held the improv sessions at set times over 2 days and invited *everyone* from *all* three intervention wards to meet in a specific room within an hour window—this would give our participants a chance to come for anywhere from 15 minutes to an hour. We used three Liberating Structures in the design of these sessions: Improv Prototyping, Fishbowl and What, So What, Now What. Improv Prototyping was the main structure, but we embedded it in a fishbowl, whereby the role playing took place in an inner circle while the outer circle observed and took notes. And we used the What, So What, Now What structure to debrief with participants about clear practices, communication patterns, and new ideas. Guidelines for all three structures can be found on the Liberating Structures website. This was the general structure of each "What if" session:

- Facilitator asks participants to name a challenge relative to HAI prevention— something that happens unexpectedly or that is overwhelming and that makes following protocol especially difficult.
- Participants volunteer to take on roles, i.e., difficult or challenging patient/family member, nurse, charge nurse, PCA, housekeeping staff, doctor.
- Facilitator explains rules: (1) we are the audience and can't talk to you unless I interject, and (2) we, as the audience, are invisible to you.
  - Draw from variations of the same activity:
      Patient not in isolation: contact isolation, airborne, or droplet isolation.
      Or use three different actors for the same what if....
- Facilitator leads debrief: What happened? What did you notice about behaviors and communication patterns? What is significant? Why? How does this change the way you see HAI/your role?

Participants responded very well to improv scenarios. These were some ideas they chose to work through:

- What if you are collecting specimens, drawing blood, and realize...

- PCA and patient transporter go in to get patient with uncontrolled HIV infection and in contact isolation for MRSA and discover he is soiled and his hand is dripping with stool…
- Confronting a colleague on something they are not doing right
- Telling visitors that children are not allowed or that only two people at a time can be in a room
- Getting a patient to sign paper: using a cheap disposable pen vs. de-germing pen vs. giving patient sanitizer foam on paper towel vs. asking patient to wear gloves vs. not setting the papers down/holding papers for patient to sign

Participants were able to draw on their experiences with relative ease. The "What if…" prompt helped them think of concrete situations when they were stuck. Through the debriefs, participants were able to empathize with each other. Following infection prevention protocol, they noted, is straightforward until…the sh*% hits the fan, literally! They remarked that they found the "What if" role playing enjoyable and useful and asked if it might be a good addition to their team meetings and huddles.

Inquiry to Action

Out of the DADs and improv sessions, new ideas emerged. Among them was the development of an infection prevention checklist for clinicians, a flashcard set for conversations with patients and their families (with visuals), and a handwashing video featuring one of the nurses washing her hands while singing happy birthday. The intervention wards were especially excited about implementing these new ideas and decided to call their initiative "Stop a Bug, Save a Life"—several names were nominated and staff from all three wards voted on their favorite (the staff members ended up really liking the process of crowdsourcing). The study team purchased bug stickers which they used to decorate their name tags, work spaces, and materials related to the study like clipboards and posters. Implementation started right away, and the study team gathered data for a little over a year (4 months of the implementation year and 9 months of follow-up).

The team found that HAI rates "decreased in both the intervention and control wards, indicating the effectiveness of system-wide aggressive hand hygiene measures" ([21], p. 7). However, the decreases in the two groups showed different patterns of decline. The control wards had a one-time, abrupt decline, whereas the intervention wards had a gradual exponential decline that ultimately decreased to a rate lower than the lowest rate for the control wards [21]. It is possible that this is due to the open dialogues around challenges and solutions that the intervention encouraged as "differences in patient safety culture over time became significantly more positive in the intervention group" [21]. Due to the experimental nature of this study, results reported are definitely on the conservative side, but the lessons we learned also provided insight into worthwhile affordances.

Similar to what occurred in the previously cited interventions at Albert Einstein and the Pennsylvania VA facilities, intervention staff commented on the fact that they were pleased to be contributors to infection prevention instead of just recipients of "yet another thing" to implement. And although the idea of horizontal problem solving was novel and took some time to get used to (roughly 3 months), conversations with the floor managers revealed that "Stop a Bug, Save a Life" brought awareness around ownership of infection prevention: "Before, staff would place blame on the patients and visitors, and now they are beginning to question, how do I contribute, which is reflexive, just like the what if sessions. They are starting to ask themselves, what if X happens, how do I handle it?" (Personal Interview, April 2012). Ward managers also commented on how refreshing the different elements of the PD approach had been, e.g., the use of role playing and naming contest, and they planned to use them for other challenges such as where to place urinals.

In some ways, even though it was a randomized controlled study and by nature scientific, "Stop a Bug, Save a Life" provided three cultural/social/relational gains:

1. Conversation between stakeholders where it didn't exist before
2. Social proof of existing, bottom-up practices and ideas and
3. Inspiration to transfer new knowledge about creative, inclusive ways to engage with other challenges

This occurred in a little over a year. Imagine these three sources of "social glue" infused into the long-term culture of a health care organization! The staff we worked with were burdened with issues of staff turnover, accreditation, and especially time. It was no wonder that they were hesitant to volunteer information initially—what if what they said got them into trouble? This work proves yet again that trust takes time. As a facilitator I learned, it also takes courage.

Concluding Thoughts: Communication and Courage

It is very easy for us to default to engrained, auto-pilot behaviors. As a patient having minor surgery on my toe, it felt better for me to not confront my doctor—at least in the moment. And as a facilitator of PD, DADs, and improv sessions, I had the desire more than once to revert to conventional interview or focus group formats when faced with no-shows, quiet participants, or contrived responses. During the study, I was not alone in my angst. One of the hospital ward managers confessed during a debrief interview: "I've learned a lot, but it's hard to hear people out. There is room for 'idiosyncrasies,' but what we do needs to be backed by evidence. I'm tempted to use discipline because it's the quickest way to effect change. This is because I am ultimately responsible for the unit" (Personal Interview, April 2012). In that conversation, we agreed that working through those old patterns also takes time—that we needed to be patient with ourselves. A month later when we met again, we touched base on challenges and insights. He mentioned that despite it seeming like it would be a waste of time, the best way for him to generate ownership and engage his staff at a deeper level was becoming through the DADs. The process was now familiar, and the staff felt safe to contribute solutions, especially in a climate of uncertainty.

In hindsight, and with the benefit of reading Brene Brown's amazing work telling us that you can't have courage without being vulnerable first, I can see how brave every person on our team had to be during the first 3 months of our study. We invited "everyone" to a kick-off meeting attended by a very small handful of stakeholders—a much smaller group than we had anticipated. We repeated DAD after DAD with little to no PD or DAD experience under our belts. We often didn't know if the information we were collecting would be useful. In other words, we lived with a general unease and often exchanged glances of, *are we remotely on track here?* But at the same time, we plowed through dialogue after dialogue. Fittingly, we walked by a lab on our way from the research building to the hospital which had a plaque above the doorframe displaying Albert Einstein's famous quote: "If we knew what we were doing, it wouldn't be called research." I'd smile every time we passed that lab.

We also did this together, and we consulted with more experienced PD practitioners, doctors, and social scientists. For many of us in leadership positions, despite working well with others, going at it alone is our default mode. Asking for help and feedback tests our courage, precisely by making us vulnerable. For many of us, getting feedback at every stage can feel inefficient. After all, over the years, we've learned to depend on ourselves, and others have learned to depend on us. But the courage to work with others makes our work even better, and it makes us even greater as leaders by reminding us that the work is bigger than any single person. As Brown reminds us, going it alone is a myth about courage.

Brown also highlights another myth: You can engineer the uncertainty and discomfort out of vulnerability. Giving the appearance of certainty is another place where leaders and Type A folks thrive. As researchers, I think we made about every attempt possible to engineer the uncertainty out of the project—that was until, as one of the ward managers put it, "the rubber hit the road." We could control the study design and the protocol, but we could never control the human factor. Imagine inviting busy people doing life or death work (literally) to an improv session! We never knew if ward staff or families would be able to make their appointments with us. There were times when we had to wait for participants to show up. And there were times when individuals eating their lunch in the break room talked with us instead. Even harder to control was the implementation of PD ideas. We had very little control on that. I say very little because it did help that the study was backed up by the health system administration and the PI was the health care epidemiologist, so the top-down element mattered. Often we think about things in binaries. They are either top-down or bottom-up. They are either a leader's work or the people's work. Engaging everyone requires the courage to step out of binaries into a messier space—where complexity lives—where you get out what you put in and where you will never be the same.

Four years ago when I was in the labor and delivery room having my daughter, the head nurse came into the room, and without washing her hands put on gloves. I said to her, "I'd really prefer it if you washed your hands before doing any work on me." She was shocked but turned around, took off her gloves, washed her hands, and put on new gloves. The other nurses were wide-eyed. I smiled and thanked her.

References

1. Westley F, Zimmerman B, Patton M. Getting to maybe: how the world is changed. New York: Random House; 2006.
2. Baxter R, Taylor N, Kellar I, Lawton R. What methods are used to apply positive deviance within healthcare organisations? A systematic review. BMJ Qual Saf. 2016;25(3):190–201. https://doi.org/10.1136/bmjqs-2015-004386.
3. Pascale R, Sternin J, Sternin M. Hospital infections: acting into a new way of thinking. In: The power of positive deviance. Boston: Harvard Business Review Press; 2010.
4. Association of State and Territorial Health Officials (ASTHO). Eliminating healthcare associated infections: state policy options. 2012. Retrieved from: http://www.astho.org/HAI_Policy_Toolkit/.
5. Cochrane AL. Effectiveness and efficiency: Random reflections on health services. Nuffield Trust. 1972. Retrived from https://www.nuffieldtrust.org.uk/research/effectiveness-and-efficiency-random-reflections-on-health-services.
6. Sackett DL, Rosenberg WM, Gray JA, Haynes RB, Richardson WS. Evidence based medicine: What it is and what it isn't. BMJ. 1996;312:71–2.
7. McCandless, K. (2012). FAQs: What traditional top-down assumptions do liberating structures challenge? Liberating Structures. Retrieved May 4, 2020 from http://www.liberatingstructures.com/faq-search/everything-you-always-wanted-to-know-abo/what-traditional-top-down-assumptions-do-liberatingstructur.html.
8. Singhal A, Bjurström E. Reframing the practice of social research: solving complex problems by valuing positive deviations. Int J Commun Soc Res. 2015;3(1):1–12.
9. Singhal A, Svenkerud P. Diffusion of evidence-based interventions or practice based positive deviations. J Dev Commun. 2019;29(2):54–66.
10. Glouberman S, Zimmerman B. Complicated and complex systems: what would successful reform of Medicare look like? Commission on the Future of Healthcare in Canada. 2002. Retrieved from: https://www.alnap.org/system/files/content/resource/files/main/complicatedandcomplexsystems-zimmermanreport-medicare-reform.pdf.
11. Lawton R, Taylor N, Clay-Williams R, Braithwaite J. Positive deviance: a different approach to achieving patient safety. BMJ Qual Saf. 2014;23(11):880–3. https://doi.org/10.1136/bmjqs-2014-003115.
12. Lipsitz L. Understanding health care as a complex system: the foundation for unintended consequences. JAMA. 2012;308(3):243–4. https://doi.org/10.1001/jama.2012.7551.
13. McDaniel R. Strategic leadership: a view from quantum and chaos theories. Healthc Manag Rev. 1997;22(1):21–37.
14. Preismeyer H, Sharp L. Phase plane analysis: applying chaos theory in health care. Qual Manag Health Care. 1995;4(1):62–70.
15. Gallup Inc. State of the American workplace report. Washington, DC: Gallup Inc.; 2017. Retrieved from: https://news.gallup.com/reports/199961/7.aspx?utm_source=SOAW&utm_campaign=StateofAmericanWorkplace&utm_medium=2013SOAWreport.
16. Gertner J. Positive deviance. The New York Times Magazine. 2008. Retrieved from: https://www.nytimes.com/2008/12/14/magazine/14ideas-section3-t-005.html.

17. Singhal A, Greiner K. Small solutions and big rewards: MRSA prevention at the Pittsburgh veterans hospitals. In: Singhal A, Buscell P, Lindberg C, editors. Inviting everyone: healing healthcare through positive deviance. Bordentown: Plexus Press; 2010.
18. Buscell P. More we than me: fighting MRSA inspires a new way of collaborating at Albert Einstein Medical Center. In: Singhal A, Buscell P, Lindberg C, editors. Inviting everyone: healing healthcare through positive deviance. Bordentown: Plexus Press; 2010.
19. McCandless K. Liberating structures: FAQs. n.d. Retrieved from: http://www.liberatingstructures.com/faq-full-text/.
20. Lipmanowicz H, McCandless K. Discovery & action dialogue. n.d. Retrieved from: http://www.liberatingstructures.com/10-discovery-action-dialogue/.
21. Sreeramoju P, Dura L, Fernandez-Rojas M, Minhajuddin A, Simacek K, Fomby T, Doebbeling B. Using a positive deviance approach to influence the culture of patient safety related to infection prevention. Open Forum Infect Dis. 2018;5(10):ofy231. https://doi.org/10.1093/ofid/ofy231.

Epilogue

Over the course of this book, we have heard from a range of experts offering their experience, insight, and perspective on the critical interface between the patient and the health care system. Appropriately and importantly, we started with the voice of our patients and acknowledged not only the challenges and fears they face, but their aspirations and expectations for a better way. We also heard from clinicians, physicians, and nurses who are expected to be the principal advocates of patients but who themselves face barriers and challenges in navigating a system and relationships where they feel control and autonomy have been lost.

A number of contributors detailed the increasingly complex landscape of delivering the highest quality and safest care. This commitment has been complicated by demands for real value, expanded access, true efficiency, and effectiveness. At the same time, we have learned about how a patient-centered focus can start us on a journey, as individuals and as an industry, to true engagement and the resolution of the disparities faced by too many of those we serve.

Whether you have read through the book cover to cover, or simply selected those contributions most compelling or relevant to your practice, we hope you feel enlightened, informed, but most of all, stimulated, and even inspired to be a force for change. Most importantly though, we hope you have come to understand that the very idea of *the* patient interacting with *the* health care system is an overly simplistic and misleading framing of the challenge. Taken together, the chapters of the book highlight that there are as many facets to our system of care delivery as there are patients themselves. Were US health care to be a monolith, addressing the problems described here would be rather simple. Instead, we need to look at our industry for what it is: a patchwork of not just providers and practices, but bureaucracies, vendors, consultants, financiers, payers, regulators, lobbyists, policymakers, and many more. Each individual and entity comes with their own passions, interests, and priorities. To that end, a truly patient-centered view will need to be re-thought and tailored at every step. To simply enhance the experience or engagement of the patient when having surgery, interacting with the nurse, or taking their medication will miss the mark and leave us all underserved.

But it is the uniqueness and diversity of our individual patients and their needs and expectations that is both our greatest challenge and our most important opportunity for improvement. Again, there is no one patient interacting with our system

© Springer Nature Switzerland AG 2020

P. V. Sreeramoju et al. (eds.), *The Patient and Health Care System: Perspectives on High-Quality Care*, https://doi.org/10.1007/978-3-030-46567-4

and services. Every patient brings not just their genes, physiology, and biology, but also their culture, their experience, their fears, their values, their character, and most of all their hopes. In appreciating this heterogeneity, and even celebrating it, we will find that not only will our approach and treatment change, but so will our definitions of success. When a health system works, it does not deliver life or death, but confidence, comfort, wellness, and joy.

The future state we envision embraces the lessons learned in these chapters but appreciates that in each case, we will need to tailor our approach to better understand and meet the needs of our patients as individuals, and not just one of many covered lives or populations at risk. Deeper understanding of our patients is at least as complex as any genetic sequence or pharmacokinetic consideration. Patient-centered care cannot be the exclusive domain of those at the bedside. Instead, we will need to invest in the means to understand and incorporate the expectations of individuals in all that we do in designing the care delivery system of the future. It is a system that is not just highly reliable, but infinitely adaptable to the needs of the next patient, and the one after him, and the one after her, and so on.

There is much at stake and we hope this book has empowered patients, stimulated investigators, inspired students, and challenged clinicians to do better. Our hope for now is that in assembling this book, we have both helped you and challenged you to think harder about the time ahead. What is the role you will play as a leader, a provider, and advocate? Our patients are counting on each of us to do our part.

Index

A

Achieving authentic engagement, 5, 6
Active engagement, 6, 14, 34
Activities of daily living (ADL's), 36
Affordable Care Act (ACA), 22, 56–58, 85, 118, 181
Affordable health insurance
  ACA, 56, 57
  Churn, 76, 77
  cost control strategies, 79
  coverage gap, 58, 59
  employer-sponsored insurance, 57
  EMTALA, 75
  federal poverty level, 58
  Government health insurance programs, 56
  health care expenditures, 71
  managed care, 77–79
  "marketplace" plans, 74, 75
  medicaid, 73
  Medicaid and Children's Health Insurance Program, 56
  medical underwriting, 57
  medicare, 74
  Medicare, Medicaid, or Children's Health Insurance Program, 58
  premium tax credits, 58, 60
  short-term plans, 59
  uncompensated care, 75, 76
  uninsured population, 76
Agency for Healthcare Research and Quality (AHRQ), 36, 37, 85, 169
All-Payer Claims Databases (APCDs), 149
Alveolar-Arterial oxygen gradient (A-a gradient), 126
American Academy of Pediatrics (AAP), 17
American College of Cardiology/American Heart Association (ACC/AHA), 125
American Geriatrics Society, 169
American Hospital Association, 73

American Nurses Association (ANA) (2015b) model, 33
American Nurses Credentialing Center (ANCC) Magnet Recognition program standards, 37
Association of State and Territorial Health Officials ASTHO, 186
Automated medication dispensing cabinets, 35–36

B

Bad Debt, 75, 76
Barcode medication administration (BCMA), 36
Barriers/obstacles to engagement, 12–16
Behavioral Risk Factor Surveillance System (BRFSS), 143
Beryl Institute, 5
Big data, 26–28
Bundled Payment Care Improvement-Advanced (BPCIA), 141, 142
Bundled Payments for Care Improvement Initiative (BPCI), 141

C

Centers for Disease Control and Prevention (CDC), 85, 186
Centers for Medicare and Medicaid Services (CMS), 17, 31, 52, 53, 74, 99, 139, 145, 155
Charity Care program, 75, 76
Children's Health Insurance Program (CHIP), 73
Churn, 76, 77
Circle of engagement, 12
Clinical decisions, 3, 28, 125, 131, 132, 150, 164, 167, 169